Evaluating Community Nursing

DATE DUE

3/10/12		
6/11/12		

GAYLORD   #3523PI   Printed in USA

For Baillière Tindall

Senior Commissioning Editor: Jacqueline Curthoys
Project Editor: Karen Gilmour
Design Direction: Judith Wright

Evaluating Community Nursing

Karl Atkin DPhil BA(Hons)
Senior Research Fellow, Ethnicity and Social Policy Research Unit, University of Bradford, UK

Neil Lunt MA BA(Hons)
Lecturer in Social Policy, School of Social Policy and Social Work, Massey University, Albany, Auckland, New Zealand

Carl Thompson DPhil BA(Hons) RGN
Research Fellow, Centre for Evidence-Based Nursing, University of York, UK

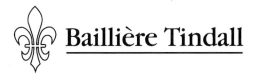 Baillière Tindall

EDINBURGH   LONDON   NEW YORK   PHILADELPHIA   SYDNEY   TORONTO   1999

Baillière Tindall
24–28 Oval Road
London NW1 7DX

The Curtis Center
Independence Square West
Philadelphia, PA 19106-3399, USA

Harcourt Brace & Company
55 Horner Avenue
Toronto, Ontario M8Z 4X6, Canada

Harcourt Brace & Company, Australia
30–52 Smidmore Street
Marrickville
NSW 2204, Australia

Harcourt Brace & Company, Japan
Ichibancho Central Building
22-1 Ichibancho
Chiyoda-ku, Tokyo 102, Japan

British Library Cataloguing in Publication Data
A catalogue record for this book is available from the British Library.

Library of Congress Cataloging in Publication Data
A catalog record for this book is available from the Library of Congress.

ISBN 0-7020-23248

Note
Medical knowledge is constantly changing. As new information becomes available,
changes in treatment, procedures, equipment and the use of drugs become necessary.
The editors, contributors and the publishers have, as far as it is possible, taken care to
ensure that the information given in this text is accurate and up-to-date. However,
readers are strongly advised to confirm that the information, especially with regard to
drug usage, complies with latest legislation and standards of practice.

The
publisher's
policy is to use
**paper manufactured
from sustainable forests**

Typeset in Malaysia
Printed in China
NPCC/01

Contents

List of contributors   vii

1. Evaluating change in community nursing   **1**
Carl Thompson, Karl Atkin, Neil Lunt

Key issues   1
Introduction   1
The structure of the book   2
The provision of community nursing   4
Evaluation and community nursing   8
Conclusion   17
Questions for discussion   17
Annotated bibliography   17

SECTION 1   EVALUATING CHANGES TO ORGANIZATIONAL CONTEXTS

**2. Addressing cultural diversities in health care – the challenge
facing community nursing**   **23**
Aliya Darr, Kuldip Bharj

Key issues   23
Introduction   23
Community nursing in a multiracial Britain   24
Equal opportunities and nurse recruitment – a development project   37
Conclusion   38
Questions for discussion   39
Annotated bibliography   40

3. Skill mix in primary care – shifting the balance   **45**
Susan Jenkins-Clarke

Key issues   45

Introduction   45
Understanding skill mix   48
The study   53
Primary care skill mix – an agenda for scrutiny   59
Conclusion   61
Questions for discussion   62
Annotated bibliography   62

4. Prescribing and community nursing – an evaluation of practice   65
Karen Luker, Lynn Austin

Key issues   65
Introduction   65
Evaluating prescribing practice   68
Implications for practice and management   73
Conclusion   74
Questions for discussion   74
Annotated bibliography   75

SECTION 2   EVALUATING CHANGES TO PRACTICE ARENAS

5. School nursing – an evaluation of policy and practice   79
Wendy Bines, Jane Lightfoot

Key issues   79
Introduction   79
Policy context   84
Policy developments and the role of the school nurse   88
Education and preparation of school nurses   97
Evaluating school nursing services   99
Conclusion   102
Questions for discussion   103
Annotated bibliography   103

6. Evaluation and community psychiatric nursing   107
Peter A. Morrall

Key issues   107
Introduction   107
Clinical autonomy   107
Research aims   108
The context of the study   109

Research methods 111
Research findings 112
Discussion 122
Conclusion 125
Questions for discussion 126
Annotated bibliography 126

7. The emergence and development of practice nursing –
implications for future policy and practice **129**
Neil Lunt, Karl Atkin

Key issues 129
Introduction 129
Evaluating the emergence and development of practice nursing 131
The policy context 131
The empirical study 134
Qualitative evaluation 135
The research findings 137
Conclusion 147
Questions for discussion 148
Annotated bibliography 149

8. Evaluating learning disability – embracing change **153**
Tony Thompson, Peter Mathias

Key issues 153
Introduction 153
The professional prerequisite 154
The historical dimension 155
Contemporary service development 156
On policy development 158
Contemporary statements relating to learning disability
nursing practice 161
Professional reaction to change 163
Questions for discussion 167
Annotated bibliography 167

SECTION 3   EVALUATING CHANGES TO PREPARATION

9. Mapping changing competences in the community adult
nursing area **171**
Annette Lankshear, Carl Tompson

Key issues 171

Introduction   171
The methodology of competence identification and examination
in community nurses   174
Establishing waymarks – the methods used   176
What did we find?   177
Horses for courses – different care settings, different skills and
competences?   178
Conclusion   190
Questions for discussion   191
Annotated bibliography   191
Appendix A   Constituents of competence groups   192

**10. Evidence-based nursing-evaluation and the role of the
community practitioner   197**
Jacqueline Droogan

Key issues   197
Introduction   197
Promoting clinical effectiveness – doing more good than harm   199
Nursing and the NHS research and development strategy   206
What can nurses do?   207
Does nursing have any research evidence?   210
Conclusion   212
Questions for discussion   213
Annotated bibliography   213

Index   215

List of contributors

Karl Atkin DPhil BA(Hons)
Senior Research Fellow, Ethnicity and Social Policy Research Unit, University of Bradford, Bradford, UK

Lynn Austin MSc RGN
Research Fellow, University of Manchester, Manchester, UK

Kuldip Kaur Bharj BSc(Hons) MSc IHSM (Cert) RSA Coun(Skills) RN RM MTD DN(Lond)
Senior Lecturer, Division of Midwifery, University of Leeds, Leeds, UK

Wendy Bines MA BA(Hons) RGN
Staff Nurse, Breast Care Unit, The General Infirmary at Leeds. Formerly Research Fellow, Social Policy Research Unit, University of York, York, UK

Aliya Darr MA BA
Research Fellow, School of Health Studies, Bradford University, Bradford, UK

Jacqueline Droogan HSc BSc RGN
Research Fellow, NHS Centre for Reviews and Dissemination, University of York, York, UK

Susan Jenkins-Clarke BSc RGN HV
Research Fellow (Nursing), Centre for Health Economics, University of York, UK

Annette J Lankshear MA BSc RGN HV
Director of Nursing Studies, University of York, Innovation Centre, York, UK

Jane Lightfoot BA CPFA
Research Fellow, Social Policy Research Unit, University of York, York, UK

Karen A Luker PhD BNurs RGN RHV NDNCert
Professor of Nursing, School of Nursing, Midwifery and Health Visiting,
University of Manchester, Manchester, UK

Neil Lunt MA BA(Hons)
Lecturer, School of Policy Studies and Social Work, Massey University,
Auckland, New Zealand

Peter Mathias PhD MSc MA BSc
Director of the Joint Awarding Bodies, London, UK

Peter Morrall PhD MSc BA(Hons) PGCE RMN RGN RNMH
Senior Lecturer, School of Health Care Studies, University of Leeds, UK

Carl Thompson DPhil BA(Hons) RGN
Research Fellow, Centre for Evidence Based Nursing, University of York, UK

Tony Thompson MA BEd(Hons) RMN DN CertEd RNT
Director, Practice Development, Ashworth Centre, Ashworth Hospital
Authority, Maghull, Liverpool, UK

1

Evaluating change in community nursing

Carl Thompson   Karl Atkin   Neil Lunt

KEY ISSUES

- Fundamental restructuring of the welfare state and the increasing importance of the nurse in these developments.
- Changing contexts for the provision of community nursing, including the increasing emphasis on primary care.
- The increasing role of the nurse in establishing health-care needs and setting priorities.
- Evaluation becomes an integral part of individual practice and service-based provision.
- Competing and complementary frameworks for evaluation are available to nurses and these include quantitative and qualitative models.

INTRODUCTION

Health care in the UK has recently undergone its most fundamental restructuring since the establishment of the postwar welfare state (Wistow et al 1994) and community nursing is at the forefront of these changes (NHS Management Executive 1993). Issues such as the introduction of contracts in health care, the separation of provision from commissioning, the increasing importance of general practice, professional training and education, needs assessment and a questioning of traditional role models are central to current policy and practice. This book makes sense of these general changes by offering an analysis of community nursing and the changing and often challenging environment within which it operates. This opening chapter explores some of the broader issues informing the provision of community nursing and outlines ways of evaluating these changes. As such the book fulfils two aims. First, it provides an empirically grounded account of community nursing and second, it illustrates the different types of evaluation available to those wishing to make sense of changes in policy and practice. However, before we discuss the broader issues raised by these two aims, we outline the structure of the book.

THE STRUCTURE OF THE BOOK

Evaluating community nursing is the focus of this book. Most existing material dealing with evaluation is informed largely by the 'medical model' and usually undertaken in acute-care settings. This text aims to take the debates about evaluation and evidence-based practice forward by applying them to community settings. Such an approach illustrates not only the complexities facing those providing and managing community nursing services but also the need to utilize a variety of evaluative strategies.

Following this introductory chapter – which explores the current changes informing community nursing and the different ways of evaluating these changes – the book is organized into three sections. The first part is concerned with the impacts of changing organizational and social contexts on nursing practice and presents empirically informed theoretical frameworks for evaluating these changing contexts. Aliya Darr and Kuldip Bharj highlight the failings of the NHS to consider ethnic diversity and pose a number of challenges that service managers need to address to ensure services are accessible and appropriate to all, within the context of a multiethnic Britain. Jenkins-Clarke's chapter describes the increasing diversity of skills within primary health-care teams and emphasizes the importance of developing evaluatory frameworks which address the new organizational contexts of 'balance' between nurses and other health-care professionals in such teams. Luker and Austin provide an exemplar for the evaluation of new and complex areas of nursing practice. Specifically, they examine the introduction of nurse prescribing in eight demonstration sites and the benefits this has brought to users and primary health-care teams.

The second part focuses on the presentation of frameworks for evaluation based around those areas of community nursing experiencing the most rapid changes: child health, community mental health, practice nursing and learning disability practitioners. Bines and Lightfoot use the example of school nursing as a case study, demonstrating the innovative ways in which practitioners have risen to the challenge of dealing with an ever more demanding population of young people. In doing so they provide valuable pointers for other practitioners to consider in the planning and evaluation of services for young people. Peter Morrall presents key findings of his evaluation of community psychiatric services. His presentation demonstrates the need for service evaluations to be flexible enough to cope with the rapidly evolving arena of mental health care in the community whilst simultaneously being able to identify the 'concealed' nature of much community mental health work. Lunt and Atkin discuss the origins of practice nurses. In adopting this historical approach, they highlight contemporary issues which will inform the development of future practice nursing services. Moreover, their qualitative approach gives a rich and contextualized picture of the current status of practice nurses within the primary health-care team. Tony Thompson and Peter Mathias also draw on historical material and theorists in their presentation of a broad framework for evaluating learning disability services. Specifically, they argue against applying unitary solutions to the complex problems of evaluating services for people with a learning disability.

The third component of the book deals with two core questions relating to individual practice. How can we approach the evaluation of groups of practitioners according to the competencies required in the unique setting of primary care? And how can individual practitioners best develop techniques which engender evaluatory skills to discrete clinical challenges? Lankshear and Thompson address the first of these questions. They present a methodological framework for service planners to apply in evaluating the competencies required of practitioners in their areas. This chapter highlights the benefits of adopting a multimethod approach to the question of evaluation in relation to community nursing. In the final chapter, Droogan implicitly recognizes the essential shift in community nursing over the past 10 years; specifically, that practitioners have developed far more professional autonomy than was ever envisaged by the profession. However, with this increased autonomy comes greater responsibility which demands new techniques of ensuring that the profession fulfils its obligation to promote optimal outcomes for the population it serves. The rise of evidence-based practice represents one way of meeting this obligation. Droogan gives practical advice on how best to begin one's professional exploration of this new area and also gives a flavour of the implications of applying such personalized evaluations of clinical solutions in key nursing topic areas such as teenage pregnancy.

Nearly all the chapters in this volume use empirical material to evaluate a particular aspect of community nursing. This emphasizes the value of evidence-based practice when discussing developments in community nursing services. However, the current rate of change in the organization and delivery of primary care sometimes means that the legislative and policy framework mentioned by some of the chapters has been superseded. Unfortunately this is inevitable in a book dealing with current issues. Nonetheless, the emphasis on the process of evaluation rather than current practice means that this does not necessarily detract from the book's general focus, particularly since each of the chapters included in this volume is informed by a similar policy context. In order to make further sense of this, it is necessary to examine the current changes informing the provision of community nursing.

THE PROVISION OF COMMUNITY NURSING

All the chapters outlined above are informed by the more general changes affecting community nursing. Following this, various interrelated themes inform the provision of community nursing. These include those of immediate relevance to community nurses, such as training, education and professional development, as well as those emerging from the general restructuring of UK health care. Each theme involves major changes in the values promoted by professionals as part of everyday service delivery. The shift from secondary care, for example, has created various opportunities for community nurses while at the same time questioning established roles and working practices. Specific issues such as skill mix, training and education and accountability have emerged as central to the management and organization of community nursing services. These debates are further informed by a general questioning of universal need and an increasing policy emphasis on priority setting in welfare provision. We now provide a necessarily brief outline of these various themes to give the reader a flavour of the wider context in which community nursing occurs.

The shift from secondary to primary care

First, and of fundamental importance to community nursing, is the shift from secondary to primary health care (Department of Health and Social Security 1987, Department of Health 1989a). This policy is not new. Since the late 1950s successive UK governments have sought to shift care from institutions to the community (Parker 1990). However, the recent policy initiatives, by emphasizing the specific importance of primary health care, introduce a broader view. Quicker hospital discharge and the growth of day surgery, as well as the more general emphasis on the care of people in their own homes for as long as possible, have established the importance of primary health care in providing community health services (Department of Health 1996a,b).

The shift to primary care creates various professional opportunities for community nurses. To take advantage of these opportunities, however, nurses will need to work more closely with general practice. The emphasis on primary health care ensures that general practice becomes the organizational base for such care. Government policy, for example, envisages 'an increasing number of general practices, through a combination of direct employment, commissioning or attachment of nurses and other professional staff, or through contracts with them, becoming a major provider of primary health care services' (NHS Management Executive 1993: p. 2). The involvement of GPs in locality commissioning and the continued existence of fundholding underwrite the importance of general practice in making decisions about the type of health care appropriate for their patient population (Goodwin 1994). The government's new White Paper further supports the role of general practice. Such decisions necessarily involve the roles of community nurses, introducing flexibility into how practices spend staffing budgets and altering the traditional relationship between GPs and community nurses (Atkin & Lunt 1996).

This changing relationship has necessitated a questioning of established roles and working practices (see Chapters 4 and 9 for examples). Current policy, for example, anticipates a more flexible nursing resource in which jobs are defined by skills rather than traditional job titles (NHS Management Executive 1993). As part of these changes we have seen a massive increase in practice nursing (see Chapter 7) and a growth in non-nursing staff offering basic care, such as venepuncture. Further, the roles of specific branches of community nursing have been the subject of considerable debate, with each profession having to justify their role in the 'new' NHS (see Chapter 5). As part of these changing roles, for example, there has been increasing policy interest in skill mix (see Chapter 3). Traditional division of labour between nurses has altered. Practice nurses, for instance, carry out work traditionally associated with district nurses and health visitors (Atkin & Lunt 1996). District nurses and health visitors, for their part, are offering a wider range of skills to meet the changing demands of general practice. The changing roles and increasing interest in skill mix have also emphasized the importance of team working among primary health-care and community-care nurses.

The interest in skill mix also raises issues about the role of training and education in ensuring nurses are adequately trained to perform the roles expected of them (UKCC 1993, 1994). Traditionally, pre- and postqualification training have ensured this. Increasingly, however, issues of skill mix, new technologies and Postregistration Education and Practice (PREP) mean that the traditional forms of training and education based on professional models are being questioned. The need to demonstrate skills and worth in both service provision and employment markets ensure that concepts of vocationalism and competence gain ground.

Establishing needs and priority setting

Debates about the role of community nurses are part of wider policy debates concerning the questioning of universal need and an increasing emphasis on priority setting. This reflects a loss of faith in traditional bureaucratic and paternalistic approaches to welfare (Hambleton 1988). As a consequence, new ways of organizing welfare provision have been sought. Two concerns, one financial and the other organizational, inform these general changes. First, government, under pressure to control public spending on health care, was concerned with using existing budgets more 'efficiently'. Consequently, 'value for money' and the inappropriate targeting of resources emerged as central aspects of government policy reports (Audit Commission 1986). Second, government policy had questioned the responsiveness and accessibility of health-care services. Griffiths' agenda for action in community care, for example, argues that community service delivery was poorly related to need (Griffiths 1988). This echoed the concerns of the earlier Audit Commission report, Community care: an agenda for action, which emphasized the importance of a flexible service response that offered a wide range of options and concluded by calling for the adjustment of services to meet the needs of people rather than the adjustment of people to meet the needs of services (Audit Commission 1986). Ensuring that provision was tailored more systematically to the assessed needs and preferences of individual users and their carers became a fundamental policy goal for future service provision. Ideals such as citizenship, consumerism, participation and choice have emerged as key policy objectives in attempts to empower recipients of health services (Department of Health 1989a, 1991).

The most obvious consequence of such policies was the introduction of markets into health care during the 1990s. These market reforms stem from the belief that two distinct functions can be identified in welfare provision – those of purchaser and provider (Pirie & Butler 1989). The purchaser's or commissioner's role involves identifying needs and setting priorities for populations. Provider organizations manage staff, respond to the needs of purchasers and provide service to meet identified priorities (Harrison 1991). Community nurses came to occupy key positions as both commissioners and providers of community nursing.

The election of the Labour government in 1997 looks unlikely to alter this basic arrangement and the separation of commissioner and provider roles will remain (Department of Health 1997). There will, however, be a subtle shift in current arrangements. For example, contracts will be replaced by longer term agreements and the rhetoric of the market is likely to be replaced by an increasing emphasis on managerialism which builds on the previous Conservative government's philosophy of managing health service resources more efficiently, while maintaining service quality. Two Audit Commission reports (1993a,b), for example, identify an important role for health commissioners in increasing the range, quality, effectiveness and responsiveness of family practice. Given this managerial incursion into professional work, nurses are expected to promote cost-effective health gains and assist in demonstrating these gains to service users, health commissioners and other professionals. This alters traditional assumptions about community nursing, with its focus on providing care for a patient (Department of Health 1996a,b).

These managerial changes have also promoted an increasing emphasis on the empowerment of users and the necessity for services to reflect their needs. Whatever the limitations of this approach (Winkler 1989), there has been greater emphasis on ensuring services are tailored to the needs of service users (see Chapter 8). The government's 1997 White Paper does nothing to alter these assumptions. Incorporating these policy aims is a major challenge with important consequences for community nursing. This emphasis has had particular relevance for the 'particular care needs' of minority ethnic groups, among others (Department of Health 1989a). There is, for example, increasing value placed on responding to the needs of people from backgrounds and cultures other than the predominantly white, middle-class make-up of the nursing profession (see Chapter 2). Community nursing is not immune from the general racism and ethnocentrism that characterizes UK welfare provision (Foster 1988, Atkin & Rollings 1993, Bowler 1994).

These changes in the management of health care have been accompanied by a recognition of health as being more than simply the absence of disease (see Chapter 5). A key policy initiative supporting this view includes the *Health of the Nation* (Department of Health 1992), and the introduction of payments and incentives in the GP contract for the provision of health promotion and chronic disease management (Department of Health 1989b). This policy emphasis on health promotion requires health professionals to have a public health agenda, to profile their populations, and to evaluate their interventions. Community nurses are expected to play a pivotal role in promoting the move to prevention.

Evaluation and evidence-based practice

This book necessarily reflects the wider policy changes outlined above. There is, however, another important aspect of the process of which this book is a part: the increasing emphasis on evaluation and evidence-based practice. To this extent, the critical and routine use of evidence as the basis for practice has emerged as a key principle of current health-care provision (see Chapter 10). This has specific implications for primary health care, often seen as a poor relation to the research priorities of the acute sector. As the Culyer Report on NHS research and development funding argues: 'It is time to place R&D in primary and community care settings on an equal footing with the acute sector' (NHS Executive 1994). More generally, the concept of evaluation in research as well as in service and professional development has become fundamental in reviewing evidence-based practice. This book not only advances this argument but also explores what is meant by evaluation. It is to this issue we now turn.

EVALUATION AND COMMUNITY NURSING

The aim of this introduction is not to baffle the reader with elaborate concepts or the theoretical juxtapositions of 'grand theorists'*. The aim is simply to outline what evaluation is; explain why it is important to community nursing; discuss some of the differences in types of evaluation; offer a methodological justification for those models of evaluation which do not 'fit' with what is sometimes held to be 'good science'; and outline what each of the chapters in this book brings to the discussion of evaluation in community nursing.

The first point to stress is that the basic idea of evaluation is nothing new to the professions. Evaluation can be simply and concisely defined as:

> *The systematic collection of information about the activities, characteristics and outcomes of programmes, personnel and products for use by specific people to reduce uncertainties, improve effectiveness and make decisions with regard to what those programmes, personnel or products are doing and affecting.* (Patton 1982: p. 15)

However, what is new – and what this definition makes explicit – is the need to be *systematic* in our efforts to collect and analyse data on how our services, professional and technical activities or simple day-to-day interactions impact on the lives of those with whom we work. It is no longer sufficient to rely on haphazard reassurances not visible to anyone other than the person doing the evaluation. To this extent, evaluation is distinct from other forms of intervention and is a systematic application of research methods around a particular programme. The other important point of evaluations is that they can be *used* both by the individual and by others facing similar problems. This in turn raises some interesting dilemmas for the professional wishing to get involved in evaluation.

Evaluation is not simply a technical exercise involving the inputting of data into some sort of methodological 'black box' and then merely reading the findings. Evaluation has always a political dimension. Minogue nicely summarizes both the problems of evaluation and also the primary reason why nurses should foster a desire to evaluate:

> *Evaluation is not merely a technical matter, nor even a question of good practice: it is, or may be, a highly political issue ... an absence of evaluation contributes further to the uncertainties and unsystematic nature of public policy.* (Minogue 1983)

---

*Such texts are available and referenced in the annotated bibliography for readers who wish to explore the concept of evaluation further.

In short, if nurses don't evaluate what they do, how can they claim to make a positive impact on the lives of the people they care for? This is not a frivolous question. It is asked in the knowledge that the delivery of community nursing services has developed tremendously over the past 20 years and must now operate in a policy climate which has seen a number of challenges to the unrivalled acceptance of the ethos of care for care's sake (see above).

As the introduction has already demonstrated, the context in which services are delivered has changed considerably over the past decade. The rise of managerialism and its associated emphasis on efficiency, effectiveness and the primacy of the 'user', as well as on decentralized decision making and greater bureaucratic autonomy, have significant implications for nursing, both in terms of changes to traditional structures of accountability and the processes which have grown in parallel with these changes. Many, if not all nurses, for instance, have at some point been involved in some form of evaluation; clinical audit, needs analysis, action research, R&D projects and service reviews all constitute forms of evaluation. This is an issue we return to later in the chapter.

Evaluating policy and practice

Community nurses play a unique role in the field of social policy, which goes far beyond the simple carrying out of directives passed down to them from above. Nurses, like other professionals involved in the delivery of welfare, make an *active* contribution to the public face of social policy. A nurse's own interpretations and actions, for example, represent the day-to-day enactment of health policy. As Lipsky states:

> In an impressive range of welfare state policies the residual discretion
> enjoyed by workers who interact with and make decisions about clients
> results in workers effectively 'making policy'. They effectively 'make policy'
> not in the sense that they articulate care objectives or develop mechanisms to
> achieve these objectives. Rather, they make policy in the sense that
> aggregation of their separate discretionary and unsanctioned behaviour
> adds up to patterned agency behaviour overall. (Lipsky 1980)

Implicit in the notion of 'street-level bureaucracy' is a recognition that policy is shaped at a number of different levels and, within these, in a number of different arenas. Given this, Gillian Fulcher (1989) provides a useful model which can be adapted for understanding the UK health-care context (Fig. 1.1). Within Fulcher's model the term 'policy levels' refers to those stages at which policy is shaped. Arenas are those areas within policy levels in which decisions are made, debates ensue and discretion exercised. Within the model the active role of the individual is recognized and, for nurses, the notion that they shape policy at a number of different levels and in a number of arenas

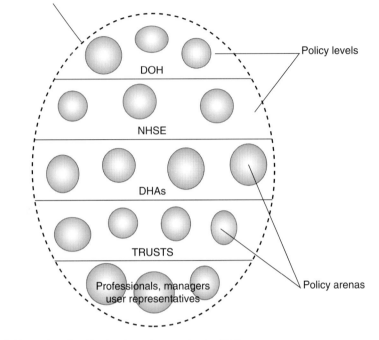

NHS apparatus, legislation, resources etc.

DOH

NHSE

DHAs

TRUSTS

Professionals, managers user representatives

Policy levels

Policy arenas

Fig. 1.1 Examples of policy levels and arenas in the NHS.

is especially pertinent. An example here might help to illustrate the point (Box 1.1).

This example highlights the multiple levels and arenas in which one professional can shape a significant contribution to local policy. Evaluation can occur at any policy level from participation in large-scale reviews of community provision through organization-wide clinical audits, down to individual reflective practice techniques.

Policy and practice: a contested domain

At a general level, despite emphasizing the role of the individual in evaluation, it is also important to recognize that policy and practice and therefore any attempt at evaluation occur within a contested domain. We have already mentioned the political dimensions of evaluation. To simply regard evaluation as a technical exercise is to miss its social, political and value orientation (Guba & Lincoln 1989). Policy, for example, cannot be wholly regarded as a 'bottom-up' approach and as we demonstrated above, community nurses have to operate within a specific policy and practice framework. Following this, evaluation has to acknowledge that there are various 'stakeholders' whose perspectives have to be taken into account when evaluating a particular

Box 1.1 Different aspects of evaluation

A district nursing team leader is asked to prepare a policy for her team's clinical supervision and to 'build in' evaluation at an early stage in order to better understand its impact on patients and the staff. Some of the areas she must take into consideration include:

◆ the variety of models of supervision in place already – this may involve negotiation and organizational change

◆ the normative models of supervision available to teams and whether these offer anything better than what is in place already – this may involve research and/or critical appraisal skills

◆ the cost-effectiveness of various options (time scales, opportunity cost: could time be better spent doing something else?) and how to establish it – this may involve liaison with external researchers such as health economists and/or other sources of advice such as the Royal Colleges

◆ the issue of implementation and how best to introduce any changes – this might involve negotiation with representatives of staff, other disciplines, training coordinators and local managers

◆ the issue of evaluation design – again she must take advice from researchers and make the design both appropriate and credible to participants and the end-users of the final report

intervention or service (Smith & Cantley 1985, Twigg & Atkin 1994). Debates about community nursing, for example, are wider than community nursing per se and reflect the interest of different stakeholders, including community nurses themselves, the GPs they work with, as well as commissioners and managers of the services provided. At a broader level, the Department of Health is central to establishing the policy and practice context within which community nursing operates. Finally, there are, of course, the needs and views of the potential or actual service users.

The perspectives of different stakeholders may not be the same and nor may a successful outcome for one stakeholder be a successful outcome for another. Evaluation must therefore recognize the multiconstituencies of social reality and that these different constituencies not only imply different interests but in some cases different interpretations of reality. Further, two different interpretations of social reality do not necessarily have the same status but occur within a power dynamic, where one account may have greater authority than others. A plurality of world views is thus possible and these views may exist within a power dynamic and have unequal possibilities of being realized. This forms the basis of a power struggle in which different world views serve to produce a 'legitimate version of the world' which is recognized by others (Bourdieu 1994). Put more simply, this approach is a reminder that policy is not just a reflection of the activities of health professionals, but represents that context in which their activities are interpreted and acted upon. For example, GPs have to act according to the specifications of their contract with the Department of Health. During the 1990s, the Department of Health wished to introduce considerable changes to this contract and despite resistance from GPs, managed to secure most of them. However, the power of the Department of Health is not absolute and general practice did win important concessions, such as the expansion in the employment of practice nurses (see Chapter 7).

Models of evaluation available to the practitioner

This chapter has so far illustrated the diversity of factors facing the practitioner considering evaluation. Practically, there are a number of different models of evaluation which the practitioner might wish to contemplate (Box 1.2).

The question of appropriateness concerns the suitability of the chosen design for the purposes of the evaluation. It is therefore important to ensure that the approach adopted is in keeping with the aims and objectives of the proposed evaluation. There is no 'gold standard' or hierarchy of evaluative approaches. Just as in other forms of research, practitioners must consider whether the stance adopted is appropriate. For example, if one wished to explore the daily life experiences of young people living with HIV in the community from their own perspective, then a survey of closed and limited response questions would not be as appropriate as a qualitative, indepth exploration of a number of individual accounts, using techniques such as depth interviewing or a form of observation.

Consequently, the practitioner must define the purposes of the evaluation and the features of the problem, service or technique under scrutiny. The chapters in this book represent a variety of responses to these questions. Some are presented as theoretical responses to practical questions such as how best to consider learning disability services given the changing nature of the service delivery context and the new groups of stakeholders – such as the voluntary sector – in the delivery of care. Others represent specific policy evaluations of school nursing, the provision of nursing services to minority ethnic groups, the role of nurse prescribing and the implications of skill mix for community nurses. Some chapters, such as the discussion of practice nursing, examine the accounts of different stakeholders.

Why should nurses consider evaluation?

There are four increasingly pressing reasons why nurses should 'do the right thing' and be prepared to examine their activities from a more systematic and

Box 1.2 Models of evaluation

Systems analysis: quantitative measurement of inputs and outputs, looking at effectiveness and efficiency

Behavioural objectives: focuses on the extent to which clear, specific and measurable goals are achieved

Needs-based: examines the extent to which actual client needs are being met

Connoisseurship: considers the extent to which the programme (or whatever is the focus) meets the evaluator's own, expertise-derived standards of excellence

Accreditation: external accreditors determine the extent to which the programme meets agreed professional standards

Adversarial: two teams of evaluators do battle over the pros and cons and the issue of whether a programme should be continued

Transaction: involves a concentration on the programme processes

Decision making: the evaluation is structured by the decisions to be made

Discrepancy: compares implementation and outcome ideals to actual achievements

Illuminative: focuses on qualitative methods, inductive analysis and naturalistic enquiry (although, as we shall argue, qualitative methods could reasonably be a component in any of the models outlined here)

Responsive evaluation: emphasizes responsiveness to all the stakeholders in evaluation

(House 1978, reproduced in Robson 1993)

critical standpoint. First, as we have seen, nurses are in a pivotal position to shape policy and for many patients they represent the public face of health services. This is a privilege but with it comes responsibility, especially as shaping policy from a position of relative ignorance is a dangerous pastime. Just as professionals acting alone can be aggregated to make up the collective face of policy in services, so can single decisions made from a position of ignorance be aggregated to make services as a whole appear unresponsive, alienating, distant and offhand.

Second, nurses are ideally placed to influence those in the various policy levels and arenas through which health policy passes. Having generally established a trust relationship with the general public, evaluation provides the opportunity for nurses to maximize such a position by influencing policy makers at the upper levels of the policy apparatus. If the nursing position can be shown to be based on something other than gut instinct or anecdote then subsequent decisions can be more easily questioned and the criterion for that questioning be made more transparent. In short, evaluation offers nurses a much stronger position in the politics of the NHS and gives their actions credibility.

Third, evaluation is part and parcel of the ethical responsibilities of the profession, not just in terms of furthering our knowledge of what might harm our clients but also in terms of the professional responsibility nurses have to each other to pass on knowledge gained through evaluation via good quality dissemination strategies. The new structures and processes associated with the implementation of the NHS research and development strategy and its links with clinical effectiveness should do much to foster this new spirit of information exchange and techniques for dissemination. Jacqui Droogan's chapter, for example, captures the essence of what such developments mean for practitioners at the front line of service delivery.

Finally, evaluation gives community nursing the ammunition to defend itself against unwarranted incursions on what it does. Just as nurses should be able to demonstrate that what they do actually has a positive impact on the lives of patients, those that seek to challenge professional intervention from alternative paradigms (such as managerialism) should also have to demonstrate that what they propose offers something equally or more beneficial to the recipients of services. For too long nurses have borne the brunt of 'service reviews', 'skill mix' and 'service developments' without the tools to question and contribute to elements of management that can have tumultuous impacts on the profession, services and, most importantly, patients. On a philosophical level, this point is another reminder that evaluation of policy and practice is a contested domain, incorporating the perspectives of different stakeholders (see above). If the profession claims that what they do is 'special' and 'unique' then evaluation is sure to be a part of this process; this book offers a starting point for practitioners, researchers and managers who are interested in moving forward in an informed and coherent fashion.

The qualitative/quantitative dilemma

Before leaving our discussion of evaluation it is important to mention another aspect of the debate: the qualitative and quantitative dilemma. The usual way of establishing the value of qualitative research in health care is by setting it up in opposition to quantitative techniques. Indeed, many accounts of qualitative research begin by discrediting quantitative techniques by describing how they devalue complexity, deny the importance of context and ignore the relevance of much research on health care in 'real' situations. Advocates of quantitative techniques, for their part, often dismiss qualitative accounts as descriptive, unsophisticated and unable to offer generalizations about the social world. Such opposition is unhelpful (McLaughlin 1991). Qualitative

methodologies are not a substitute for quantitative ones; they are complementary. Both research methods can provide valuable insights and it is not a
question of either/or but using the most appropriate methodology to answer
the research question. As with evaluation, there is no 'gold standard' or most
desirable methodology on which to base evaluation.

However, traditionally evaluative studies have not used qualitative
methodologies. Qualitative approaches were somehow seen as 'non-scientific',
small-scale studies from which it was impossible to generalize. Limited ideas
about what constitutes 'proper' science may, however, affect whether the
potential of qualitative research within evidence-based health care can be
realized. Good qualitative research still has to follow a logical, rigorous
methodology. It is certainly not a question of making it up as you go along.
The techniques of carrying out a qualitative study are, of course, different
from quantitative techniques. There is, for example, less concern with hypo-
thesis testing and large sample sizes and more of an emphasis on understanding subject meanings in their social context (Mishler 1986). This, however,
does not belittle the role of qualitative work. Good qualitative research works
to a set of aims and objectives, follows a clear method of sampling, data
collection and analysis, locates findings within the wider literature and draws
conclusions. This, of course, is similar to quantitative methods. In effect, the
real distinction is between 'good' and 'bad' research.

In this respect there is an urgent need to develop accessible methods for
critical appraisal of qualitative research reports (Britten 1996). Were the right
research questions asked? What was the sample strategy? How was the
adequacy of theory, data collection and analysis ensured? One would, of
course, ask these questions about a paper based on quantitative techniques.
It is no use trying, however, to judge qualitative research on the criteria
of quantitative research or indeed vice versa. This is where the opposition
we mentioned earlier emerges. The most important measure of standards in
qualitative research is whether the knowledge produced by the research
incorporates an understanding of subjective meanings within their social
context.

The value of qualitative approaches

Qualitative research begins by accepting that there are different ways of
making sense of the world and consequently is concerned with eliciting the
meanings ascribed by different social actors (Gubrium & Silverman 1989). It is
not concerned with the situation before and after an intervention but more
interested in what goes on during the intervention; in other words, understanding what is in the 'black box' rather than simple inputs and outcomes
(Morse 1994). This approach is highly valuable when using research findings
to inform policy and practice.

◆ Such an approach highlights patients' social contexts and their perceptions of the appropriateness of treatment and care.
◆ Qualitative techniques emphasize the importance of understanding the social processes involved in the management of clinical change and service development.
◆ Qualitative approaches enable the perspectives of different stakeholders to be understood and located within a wider empirical framework. This goes beyond simple description.

Evaluations of drug therapy reflect the particular strengths of how qualitative research studies can supplement those grounded in more 'scientific' approaches such as the randomized controlled trial. For example, the clinical effectiveness of a drug can be well established during drug trials. This, however, is not the end of the story. Patients might find the medication distasteful, inconvenient and cumbersome to take. Non-compliance could therefore be a problem. Management might be concerned about the cost and long-term benefit of medication. Health professionals might have their own 'pet' ways of treating people and as a consequence be reluctant to use the new medication. Qualitative research can help uncover these different accounts and ensure more effective policy and practice.

The value of quantitative methods

Having established the value of qualitative research in evaluation, it is perhaps important to remind the reader of the value of quantitative approaches. We make no apologies for beginning with a justification of qualitative methodologies because these are – undeservedly – seen as having little relevance for evaluative studies. However, to avoid contributing to the unhelpful opposition between quantitative and qualitative techniques mentioned earlier, it is useful to present an account of the benefits and pitfalls of quantitative techniques.

Social research and research into social phenomena (for they are not always the same thing!) rely on achieving a balance between four competing philosophical challenges – understanding, explanation, individualism and holism (Holliss 1996). Whilst qualitative techniques offer valuable models for exploration and hence understanding and can cope with the complexity of the social world by taking a holistic view, they rarely offer the chance to generalize to whole populations. Quantitative methods, on the other hand, are ideally suited to the tasks of explanation and the interplay between limited numbers of identified variables. They look at causal relationships and associations and offer the possibility, if conducted correctly, of generalizing to whole populations.

Neither method is better than the other and the rules of application are not cast in stone. The key to successful evaluation lies in the concept of appropriateness. For example, there would be little value in adopting a solely qualitative approach to evaluating the physical impact of a newly introduced dressing for leg ulcers. The desire here is to explain which dressing or technique provides the optimal result. The approach needs to be comparative and we need to apply the findings to other patients as part of the change in practice implied by undertaking the evaluation in the first place. Clearly, in this case, some form of controlled trial using statistical analysis of the results would be an 'appropriate' response. We may wish to combine the results of the trial with qualitative data about the experience of the two groups using the new dressings in order to offer further insight and help inform the practice change. Again, this would be an appropriate course of action.

CONCLUSION

Health care in the UK, like other forms of welfare provision, is undergoing its most fundamental restructuring for 50 years. Community nursing is at the forefront of these changes and as a consequence has found its traditional role and practices questioned. This book addresses these changes by offering an analysis of community nursing, while at the same time outlining the evaluative tools necessary to facilitate this analysis. In doing so, the book takes forward the debates on community nursing provision, evidence-based practice and evaluative strategies.

QUESTIONS FOR DISCUSSION

◆ How do you currently evaluate practice in your service?

◆ Does this evaluation *impact* on your service?

◆ How appropriate are the methods of evaluation you use? (do you match the methods to the questions on which you base the evaluation?)

◆ Are there parts of your role which you feel are not amenable to evaluation and why?

ANNOTATED BIBLIOGRAPHY

Robson C 1993 Real world research: a resource for social scientists and practitioner-researchers. Blackwell, London

In this text Colin Robson provides an excellent overview of research methods, techniques and strategies. Of particular interest to readers of this text will be the section on designing evaluations (pp. 170–186). He deals with this sometimes complex area with great aplomb and makes it readable at the same time.

House E R 1978 Assumption underlying evaluation models. Educational Researcher 7: 10–12

This is essential reading for any serious student of evaluation – a seminal paper and an interesting historical note.

Morse J (ed) 1994 Critical issues in qualitative research methods. Sage, London

This is a methodologically comprehensive text relating specifically to nursing and with enough depth to satisfy full-time researchers and practitioners alike. Readers should pay particular attention to the chapter by Swanson and Chapman (pp. 66–93) on qualitative evaluation.

Crombie I K with Davies H T O 1996 Research in health care: design, conduct and interpretation of health services research. Wiley, Chichester

This is a useful thumbnail guide to the various strategies available to the budding research/evaluation designer. Whilst most of the designs are more suited to quantitatively 'appropriate' problems there is a small section on the value of qualitative techniques. Overall, Crombie provides a very readable work, grounded firmly in the NHS.

REFERENCES

Atkin K, Lunt N 1996 Negotiating the role of the practice nurse in general practice. Journal Of Advanced Nursing 24: 498–505

Atkin K, Rollings J 1993 Community care in a multi-racial Britain: a critical review of the literature. HMSO, London

Audit Commission 1986 Making a reality of community care. HMSO, London

Audit Commission 1993a Practice makes perfect: the role of the family health service authority. HMSO, London

Audit Commission 1993b Their health, your business: the new role of the district health authority. HMSO, London

Bourdieu P 1994 Distinction: a social critique of taste. Routledge, London

Bowler I 1994 They're not the same as us: midwife stereotypes of South Asian maternity patients. Sociology of Health And Illness 15 (2): 151–178

Britten N 1996 Qualitative interviews in medical research. In: Mays N, Pope C Qualitative research in health care. BMJ Publishing, London

Department of Health and Social Security, Welsh Office, Northern Ireland Office and Scottish Office 1987 Promoting Better Health, Cmnd 249. HMSO, London

Department of Health 1989a Caring for people, Cmnd 849. HMSO, London

Department of Health 1989b General practice in the National Health Service: the 1990 contract. HMSO, London

Department of Health 1991 The Citizen's Charter: raising the standard, Cmnd 1599. HMSO, London

Department of Health 1992 The health of the nation: a strategy for health in England. HMSO, London

Department of Health 1996a Primary care: delivering the future. HMSO, London

Department of Health 1996b Choice and opportunity: primary care – the future. HMSO, London

Department of Health 1997 The new NHS. HMSO, London

Foster M C 1988 Health visitors' perspectives on working in a multi-racial society. Health Visitor 61: 275–278

Fulcher G 1989 Disabling policies? A comparative approach to education policy and disability. Falmer Press, London

Goodwin S 1994 Effective purchasing of community nursing, Liverpool: Mersey RHA and Mersey Regional Association of Fundholding Practices

Griffiths R 1988 Community care: an agenda for action. HMSO, London

Guba E G, Lincoln Y S 1989 Fourth generation evaluation. Sage, London

Gubrium J F, Silverman D 1989 The politics of field research: sociology beyond enlightenment. Sage, London

Hambleton R 1988 Consumerism, decentralisation and local democracy. Public Administration 66: 125–147

Harrison S 1991 Working The Market: Purchaser/Provider Separation In English Health Care. International Journal Of Health Services 21 (4): 625–635

Holliss M 1996 The philosophy of social science. In: Bunnin N, Tsui-James E P (eds) The Blackwell companion to philosophy. Blackwell, London

House E R 1978 Assumption underlying evaluation models. Educational Researcher 7: 10–12

Lipsky M 1980 Street level bureaucracy: dilemmas of the individual in public service. Russell Sage, New York

McLaughlin E 1991 Oppositional poverty: the quantitative/qualitative divide and other dichotomies. Sociological Review 39 (2): 292–308

Minogue W J D 1983 Adventures in curriculum. Allen and Unwin, Sydney

Mishler E G 1986 Research interviewing: context and narrative. Harvard University Press, Cambridge

Morse J (ed) 1994 Critical issues in qualitative research methods. Sage, London

NHS Executive 1994 Supporting research and development in the NHS: the report of a task force led by Professor Anthony Culyer. HMSO, London

NHS Management Executive 1993 Nursing in primary health care: new world, new opportunities. HMSO, London

Parker G 1990 With due care and attention. Family Policy Studies Centre, London

Patton M Q 1982 Practical evaluation. Sage, Newbury Park and London

Pirie M, Butler E 1989 Extending care. Adam Smith Institute, London

Robson C 1993 Real world research: a resource for social scientists and practitioner-researcher. Blackwell, London

Smith G, Cantley C 1985 Assessing health care: a study in organisational evaluation. Open University Press, Milton Keynes

Twigg J, Atkin K 1994 Carers perceived: policy and practice in informal care. Open University Press, Buckingham

United Kingdom Central Council (UKCC) 1993 The future of professional practice and education. UKCC, London

United Kingdom Central Council (UKCC) 1994 The future of professional practice: the Council's standards for education and practice following registration. UKCC, London

Winkler F 1989 Consumerism in health care: beyond the supermarket model. Policy and Politics 15 (1): 1–18

Wistow G, Knapp M, Hardy B, Allen C 1994 Social care in a mixed economy. Open University Press, Buckingham

Section 1

Evaluating changes to organizational contexts

2. Addressing cultural diversities in health care –
the challenge facing community nursing   *23*

3. Skill mix in primary care –
shifting the balance   *45*

4. Prescribing and community nursing –
an evaluation of practice   *65*

2

Addressing cultural diversities in health care – the challenge facing community nursing

Aliya Darr   Kuldip Bharj

KEY ISSUES

◆ The British population now consists of people from a diverse range of ethnic, cultural and religious backgrounds.

◆ There is increasing pressure on the NHS to provide equitable, accessible and culturally sensitive health services.

◆ The failure to employ a multicultural workforce limits the ability of the NHS to adequately address the health needs of minority ethnic communities.

◆ The recruitment of South Asians into the nursing profession is a serious problem.

INTRODUCTION

Over the past two decades community nursing has undergone considerable reforms largely as a result of changes in health policy, clinical practice and nurse education (Koch 1994). During this period major demographic changes have also taken place, affecting the socioeconomic structure of Britain's population as well as the nature of its health needs. There now exists a plethora of different and diverse minority ethnic communities, providing a major challenge for the NHS. There has, however, been increasing criticism of the NHS in terms of its ability to identify and address the health needs of Britain's minority ethnic communities in an equitable and appropriate manner (Rudat

1994, Balarajan & Raleigh 1995). In particular, health professionals have failed to prioritize the health problems and concerns of disadvantaged groups. This has ensured that the needs of minority ethnic communities have remained largely unaddressed (GLARE 1987, NAHA 1988).

A major challenge facing the nursing profession in its efforts to address the needs of a multiethnic society is the need to employ a more culturally diverse workforce. The failure to attract people from minority ethnic backgrounds into the nursing field has been a serious cause for concern for the NHS (Akinsanya 1988, Bharj 1995). Despite growing evidence suggesting this trend is worsening, little effort has been made to investigate these low rates of recruitment by either educational institutions or local NHS Trusts (Beishon et al 1995, Gerrish et al 1996).

In this chapter we critically evaluate community nursing's efforts to provide culturally appropriate and accessible services, before focusing on the specific issues of nurse recruitment and retention among minority ethnic populations. The chapter is in two parts. First, it sets out the policy framework which informs nursing practice and assesses how useful guidelines have been in enabling health professionals, and in particular nurses, to deliver culturally sensitive and responsive health care services. By drawing upon specific empirical examples, it will also highlight some of the common issues and concerns which confront nursing professionals working within multiethnic settings.

Second, the chapter examines equal opportunities and employment in the NHS. It focuses particularly on the problem of nurse recruitment by outlining a research and development project currently being undertaken at Bradford University*. This project is of interest not only because it aims to explore the wide-ranging factors which deter South Asians from pursuing careers in health care, but also because it sets out an agenda for institutional change aimed at improving recruitment practice. As such, it illustrates the value of practical action informed by a critical evaluation of the problems involved.

COMMUNITY NURSING IN A MULTIRACIAL BRITAIN

The presence of minority ethnic groups in Britain

According to the 1991 census, there are approximately three million people from minority ethnic groups in Britain, constituting approximately 6% of the total population (Coleman & Salt, 1995). Statistics indicate the geographical

---

*This two-year project is a collaborative venture between the School of Health Studies at Bradford University, Bradford Hospitals NHS Trust, Bradford Community Health NHS Trust and Airedale NHS Trust. It has been funded by the West Yorkshire Education and Training Consortium.

Table 2.1 Resident population by ethnic group, Great Britain 1991

Ethnic group	Number (thousands)	Proportion of total pop (%)
White	51,874	94.5
Black, Caribbean	500	0.9
Black, African	212	0.4
Black, other	178	0.3
Indian	840	1.5
Pakistani	477	0.9
Bangladeshi	163	0.3
Chinese	157	0.3
Other, Asian	198	0.4
Other, non-Asian	290	0.5

Source: 1991 Census, Local Base Statistics, ONS Crown Copyright

distribution of people from these groups is highly uneven, accounting for up to 60% of the population in some parts of the country. As Table 2.1 highlights, people of Indian origin constitute the largest minority ethnic group in Britain today although the Caribbean, Pakistani and African populations also have a significant presence.

Identifying the health needs of minority ethnic groups

Evidence suggests there are distinct variations in both health status and access to health services amongst minority ethnic communities in comparison to the indigenous population (Townsend & Davidson 1982, Nazroo 1997). A number of studies have highlighted that people from minority ethnic groups suffer from poorer general health than their white counterparts and are more likely to develop certain conditions and illnesses (Marmot et al 1984, Rudat 1994, Balarajan & Raleigh 1995). For example, mortality rates of liver cancer, ischaemic heart disease, strokes and diabetes are much higher amongst minority ethnic groups (Balarajan & Bulusu 1990). Mortality and perinatal mortality rates are also higher for infants of mothers born outside the United Kingdom (Balarajan & Raleigh 1995). Conversely, it is evident that respiratory illnesses such as bronchitis, asthma, emphysema and pneumonia are more prevalent amongst the indigenous population (Nazroo 1997).

Not only do health variations exist between minority ethnic groups and the indigenous population, there are also clear differences in health patterns between minority ethnic groups themselves (Rudat 1994, Nazroo 1997). For example, it is apparent that Pakistanis and Bangladeshis suffer from much higher rates of coronary heart disease and diabetes than Indians and African Asians as well as the indigenous population. Similarly, rates of hypertension are much higher amongst Afro-Caribbean people than in any other ethnic group (Nazroo 1997).

At policy level there has been an increased recognition of the need to address the specific health problems faced by members of minority ethnic groups. In particular, the NHS and Community Care Act, and the policy and practice guidance associated with it, is heralded as a particularly significant piece of legislation giving clear signals to professionals working within health and social services departments to take account of the multiracial, multiethnic nature of their clients (Box 2.1).

The need to address the health needs of minority groups was again brought to the fore by the government's Health of the Nation strategy (Department of Health 1992). This stressed the importance of tackling health inequalities amongst disadvantaged groups in order to improve the health status of the population as a whole. In addition to this, the implementation of the Patient's Charter reflects a continuing commitment to health services being more responsive to the diverse needs of a multicultural society. The Charter emphasizes the requirement that health service provision must show 'respect for privacy, dignity, religious and cultural beliefs' (Department of Health 1991, amended 1995). This desire to promote a greater accountability to clients also underlines recent health care reforms which have placed a greater onus on health commissioners to encourage communities to have a voice in the way in which services are delivered through greater involvement in service planning and provision.

Arguably these changes provide the potential to veer away from the uniformity of the past which has hindered the development of appropriate health care services for minority ethnic groups. However, it is apparent that the needs of disadvantaged groups continue to be neglected as many service providers are still constrained by wider organizational priorities and resource considerations. Walker & Ahmad (1994) point to the difficulties of administering effective community care services for the more vulnerable groups in society amidst a climate of shrinking financial resources and growing suspicion

---

Box 2.1 NHS and Community Care Act 1990

◆ Identifies people from minority ethnic communities as having 'particular care needs' which require specific attention

◆ Places great emphasis on the role of professionals working in the community to strive for greater empathy with patients from different cultural and religious backgrounds

◆ Advocates a better understanding of the social circumstances of patients and their families

◆ Promotes greater involvement of minority ethnic communities in planning culturally appropriate services

of government welfare policies. Furthermore, many service providers have found that the emphasis placed on redirecting resources on the basis of need has overlooked the question of whether disadvantaged groups such as minority ethnic communities are adequately equipped to respond and benefit from these new service arrangements. So despite the widespread adoption of policy initiatives and rhetoric claiming greater choice and equity, Britain's health care services continue to be denounced for being ethnocentric and inappropriate to the needs of people from minority cultures (Cartwright 1979, Larbie 1985, Pearson 1985, Phoenix 1990). The persistence of factors such as institutional racism, discriminatory practices and lack of genuine commitment to equal opportunities has meant that many service providers are still not fully in tune with the needs of their local minority ethnic populations.

For nurses working in the community the challenge of providing effective health care has never been more important. Services previously provided in the hospital setting are increasingly being transferred into the community. Community nurses, therefore, are increasingly at the forefront of planning and delivering quality health care services to populations varying considerably in terms of ethnicity, language, culture and religion. To prepare nurses for work with such heterogeneous populations, the United Kingdom Central Council for Nursing, Midwifery and Health Visiting emphasizes the need to:

> *recognize and respect the uniqueness and dignity of each patient and client and respond to their need for care, irrespective of their ethnic origin, religious beliefs, personal attributes, the nature of their health problems or any other factors.* (Item 7, UKCC 1992)

These guidelines are especially pertinent for nurses working in community settings, who are increasingly likely to provide nursing care and develop closer links with clients from different cultural backgrounds to themselves. Working in multicultural settings also means that these nurses are more likely to encounter individuals and groups suffering from health conditions and health-related problems which they may not have experienced amongst the indigenous population. It is therefore apparent that nurses working in the community need to develop relevant skills and knowledge that enable them to provide high standards of individualized patient care. However, it is less clear how nurses, both as individuals and as members of primary health care teams, can ensure that such care is provided in an equitable and non-discriminatory manner.

Understanding the role of culture in health care

Nurses are often apprehensive about obtaining information on the cultural background of patients and worry that they are unable to learn enough about the cultures of all the ethnic groups with whom they work. Baxter (1988b), for example, found that there were a number of issues on which nurses lacked knowledge but were concerned to learn more about. These ranged from aspects of religion and dietary restriction to perceptions of hygiene and grooming practices. Not being equipped with basic information relating to different religious and cultural practices makes it easier for health professionals to make assumptions about their clients' needs and preferences based on inaccurate generalizations and stereotypes (Baxter 1988b). Midwives and health visitors are amongst those who routinely use stereotypes to make judgements about the behaviour and care needs of clients from minority ethnic backgrounds (Foster 1988, Bowler 1993a). Bowler's small-scale study, for instance, examined the ways in which midwives routinely categorized their South Asian clients as forming a group which was 'all the same' but 'not like us'. Typical views held by these midwives about the South Asian mothers they met ranged from the latter's tendency to 'make a fuss about nothing' to them 'lacking normal maternal instincts'. Furthermore, it was strongly felt by midwives in the study that these specific characteristics could be attributed to the cultural backgrounds of these women.

A number of writers have highlighted how this undue emphasis on the role of 'culture' in explaining patterns of health and health-related behaviour is simplistic and unwarranted (Ahmad 1996b, Atkin & Rollings 1993). These writers argue that this diverts attention away from other structural factors which impact upon health status with equal significance. In this way, they claim that behavioural patterns and health of minority ethnic communities can be better understood if due consideration is given to the type of housing in which they live, their level of income and the degree of awareness they hold about available services. Following this, it has been argued that over-reliance on cultural explanations has severely limited the effectiveness of health professionals to tackle the genuine and varied health needs of these minority ethnic groups. By routinely engaging in 'cultural reductionism' many service providers have been allowed to unashamedly lay the blame on communities themselves for the prevalence of health problems and diseases. Government initiatives such as the 'Stop the Rickets' and the 'Asian Mother and Baby' campaigns have both been cited widely to illustrate the way in which aspects of 'Asian culture' were perceived as problematic and in need of change (Donovan 1984, Rocheron 1988).

Health professionals, then, should consider carefully the ways in which 'culture' is used to explain health-related beliefs and patterns of behaviour. They must avoid the tendency to reify culture as something which is static and inflexible and which only has relevance to the lives of minority ethnic groups. Rather, they should look upon the way in which everyone's lives are influenced by their cultural background: culture is reflected in such basic practices as the clothes we wear and the food we eat. Looking at culture in this way should also help us to appreciate the ways in which cultural behaviour and practices naturally change over time. This is most clearly illustrated by the way in which strong kinship relationships and networks – commonly thought to characterize South Asian communities – have weakened over time (Ahmad 1996a). An increasing number of studies now reveal how families are often denied much-needed services as a result of misconceptions amongst mainstream service providers about the extent of informal care provided within Asian families (Woollett & Dosanjh-Matwala 1990a). For example, in Shah's study of Asian families with a disabled child, it was found that service providers often had the impression that all Asian families were self-sufficient and would therefore have the resources available to 'look after their own' (Shah 1992). However, Shah found – contrary to the views of service providers – that families suffered considerable isolation and frustration as a result of poor access to community nursing services and other community-based services. Clearly, cultural stereotypes about the role of family support in South Asian families have legitimated the lack of recognition of need, therefore denying the availability of much-needed services to members of disadvantaged groups.

Interpreting difference as deviance

The NHS has been slow in developing an organizational culture which is responsive to increasingly different and diverse health needs (NAHA 1988). Until the 1980s there were only limited efforts to promote equal opportunities in the provision and delivery of health services. It was generally assumed that minority groups would integrate and make use of preexisting health services (Williams 1989). These misconceptions were strengthened by the widespread belief that the availability of universal services for everyone would ensure that services were being provided in an equitable way.

The inability of the NHS to consider the nature of changes required to provide equitable provision has meant that members of minority groups continue to be disadvantaged with regard to the quality of care they receive. The persistence of institutional discrimination means that the specific requirements of minority groups are still overlooked by mainstream service providers within health and social services. For example, relatively few resources are spent on targeting the specific health concerns of minority ethnic groups, such as screening programmes for sickle cell and thalassaemia (Torkington 1991), genetic conditions affecting significant numbers of Cypriot, South Asian and Afro-Caribbean people in Britain. The failure of the NHS to prioritize resources has resulted in patchy and *adhoc* service provision for sufferers and their families, with consequences ranging from limited informed choice to avoidable suffering, stress and in some cases death (Anionwu 1993). This is in contrast to the availability of screening facilities on offer to all newborn babies for much rarer conditions such as cystic fibrosis and phenylketonuria (Chevannes 1991).

The tendency to organize service provision around white norms is reflected in the ways in which a wide spectrum of health and social services are planned and delivered (Butt & Mirza 1996). Limited progress has been made in identifying whether mainstream services are adequately addressing the needs of minority ethnic groups, particularly amongst their older populations (Blackmore & Boneham 1994). This means that services such as day centres and residential homes cater largely for the interests and needs of the indigenous population in terms of the activities they provide, the staff they employ and even the food they serve. It is not surprising, then, that few of these centres are attended by elderly people from minority groups.

This same ethnocentric model of service delivery is also used within the health service to determine the way in which clients are diagnosed. In the field of mental health, professionals are slowly beginning to acknowledge that Western ideologies of well-being and ill health may not be appropriate in assessing mental health problems amongst different cultural groups. Badger et al (1990) highlight the complexity of the situation:

> There can be problems in assessing the mental competence of people whose culture, mother tongue and life experiences may be different from those of the assessor. (p. 87)

The failure to examine what constitutes mental well-being and ill health within different cultural contexts greatly impedes the ability of practitioners to develop alternative diagnostic criteria for clients from minority ethnic backgrounds. It has been argued that until efforts are made towards acquiring better understanding of the transcultural aspects of mental illness, the danger of misdiagnosis and incorrect treatment of individuals belonging to minority cultures will continue to persist (Beliappa 1991).

Insensitive and inappropriate care

Numerous studies suggest that community health services offered to minority ethnic groups are often inappropriate and less sensitive than those offered to the indigenous population (PCHC 1992, Combes & Schonueld 1992, LFHSA 1992, Atkin & Rollings 1993, Department of Health 1993b, Ullah 1994). For example, claims are often made that women from minority ethnic communities do not make use of available community health services such as breast-screening facilities and antenatal classes. At the same time, however, little effort is made to ensure that health services are provided in an appropriate and accessible manner to all sections of the community. Indeed, in many cases people from minority communities do not even know that certain health services exist. This, of course, leads to a low uptake of these services (Atkin et al 1989). Further, once people are made aware of the range of community services on offer they show a genuine interest in using them (Badger et al 1990).

The mere availability of services, therefore, does not necessarily ensure they will be used by minority groups. Providing services in culturally sensitive and appropriate ways, however, will encourage greater utilization and at the same time promote a better image of the NHS. Unfortunately, there are many reports of harrowing experiences suffered by clients as a result of culturally insensitive treatment. Practices such as the refusal of the option to see a female doctor and the fitting of intrauterine contraceptive devices in the presence of male medical students are reported examples which Asian women have found extremely distressing. This type of insensitivity reinforces the need for health professionals to actively create environments which promote responsive and flexible health care services, built upon respect for individual preference and need.

Within the community, nurses may be aided in their work by understanding the role of support structures and specialized services for certain minority ethnic groupings. These types of organizations tend to be located in the voluntary sector and have often come into being through the efforts of community members who have identified gaps in mainstream service provision. They are often poorly resourced in terms of staff and finances and tend to survive on short-term funding, effectively limiting the type and range of services they can offer (Atkin & Rollings 1993, Watters 1996). Nonetheless, voluntary sector organizations play key roles in the lives of many disadvantaged people from minority ethnic backgrounds, providing much-needed support, advice and care to people suffering from a wide range of health and social problems. Whilst professionals working within the community should be aware of and, where necessary, refer clients to such groups, it is important to recognize their limitations. All too often mainstream organizations feel that the mere existence of specialist services within the voluntary sector absolves them of responsibility to ensure the services they provide are culturally sensitive and appropriate.

Communication and language barriers

Issues of communication and language are seen as the biggest challenge encountered by nurses in the provision and delivery of health care to minority ethnic groups (Foster 1988, FHSA 1992, Department of Health 1993a,b, Ullah 1994). Patients' testimonies also acknowledge the difficulties caused by language barriers and the negative effects these have on their experience of services (Woollett & Dosanjh-Matwala 1990a,b).

When dealing with patients who are unable to speak English fluently, difficulties arise in trying to assess whether information is conveyed effectively and patients are satisfied with the quality of care received. Bowler (1993b) found women with limited knowledge of English felt humiliated and angry at the way in which they were treated by staff who characterized them as unresponsive, rude and unintelligent. Similarly, non-English speaking parents experience particular difficulties in finding out about the existence of services for themselves and their families (Faden 1991, Shah 1992). Indeed, having access to information is a vital component in enabling clients to make informed choices about their health needs. For people whose first language is not English the ability to be assertive and exercise choice over the type of care received is very difficult if they are not aware of their rights as service users (Beech 1991, Murphy & Clark 1993). This often leads to feelings of frustration and negativity amongst patients; feelings which are compounded if they do not have access to health professionals with whom they can communicate.

In a strategic attempt to eradicate the linguistic and communication barriers faced by non-English speaking patients, numerous NHS trusts have employed a range of bilingual specialist workers. Interpreters, advocates and link workers have all been employed in areas where take-up of services amongst minority groups has been low (Baxter 1997). Not only have these workers been invaluable in bridging language barriers experienced in various health settings, they have also encouraged people from local communities to learn more about issues relating to their health and at the same time increased their satisfaction with services (Anionwu 1993).

However, despite recognition of the usefulness of interpreters in improving service provision and client satisfaction, evidence suggests that demand far outstrips supply and that within the NHS interpreting services are being merely sustained rather than developed (Baxter 1997). Indeed, in many areas where minority ethnic groups are numerically insignificant there is even less likelihood that any form of language support will be available. If clients from these communities are not fluent in English, they may often resort to using family members as interpreters which can often be highly inappropriate in situations requiring sensitivity. Even when interpreter support is available, problems can still occur if health professionals have not received training enabling them to work effectively with interpreters and do not fully understand how to control the interaction between themselves, the interpreter and the client (Shackman 1984).

More generally, it is a community nurse's responsibility to show sensitivity to the linguistic and communication difficulties faced by members of minority ethnic communities. Nurses need to ensure they are able to communicate effectively with all their client groups and that in turn clients are confident about asking questions and seeking advice. This does not necessarily require that both nurse and client speak the same language but it does mean that nurses should be sensitive to the communication process between themselves and clients from different cultural backgrounds. To this end, it is imperative that in their encounters with clients from minority ethnic backgrounds, nurses take particular care to ensure they create an environment of mutual understanding in which language is not a barrier to communication. Many health-related resources are now available in a variety of languages, mainly in leaflet form and to a lesser extent as audio and video tapes. These types of materials are widely used by health professionals within community settings to convey health education messages to specific linguistic groups on subjects as diverse as antenatal care and coronary heart disease, diabetes and disability (HEA 1994).

The need for a multiethnic nursing workforce

Employing a culturally diverse nursing workforce partially resolves some of the problems experienced by the NHS in providing responsive and accessible health care (King Edward's Hospital Fund for London 1990, Department of Health 1993a). There is a greater likelihood that such a workforce will be equipped with the appropriate skills and knowledge to deliver services in a more culturally sensitive manner. In 1993, the Department of Health published a report entitled Ethnic Minority Staff in the NHS: A Programme of Action. This acknowledged the underrepresentation of staff from minority ethnic backgrounds within the NHS (Box 2.2). The report stressed the need to eradicate discriminatory practices which deny equal opportunities to minority ethnic people seeking employment and developing a career within the NHS. Nursing was identified as presenting particular problems given the underrepresentation of staff from minority ethnic backgrounds.

Nursing and minority ethnic groups

Great efforts were made in the 1960s to recruit health professionals into the NHS from various Commonwealth countries. During this period large numbers of overseas nurses as well as ancillary workers and doctors were needed as a consequence of staff shortages (Doyal et al 1981). Evidence suggests, however, that once these nurses arrived to take up employment, they were subject to a wide range of discriminatory practices (Akinsanya 1988, Baxter 1988a, Lee-Cunin 1989). A high proportion of them were channelled into enrolled nursing training (SEN) whilst their white counterparts with equivalent qualifications were encouraged to become more prestigious, better paid, state-registered nurses (SRN). This had the effect of limiting overseas nurses' professional advancement and keeping them in low-status positions of subservience (Pearson 1987). Further, many of them were forced to work in

Box 2.2 NHS Programme of Action

1. **Recruitment and selection**
   NHS trusts and health authorities to include in their business plans a local objective to increase the proportion of minority ethnic staff in areas and grades where they are underrepresented, within a specified time scale, until fair representation is achieved.

2. **Staff development**
   To maximize the skills and potential of all personnel in a multiracial NHS workforce, with particular emphasis on the identifiable needs of people from minority ethnic groups.

3. **Racial harassment**
   To ensure NHS workplaces are free from harassment and discrimination, including racial harassment.

4. **Appointment to NHS boards**
   To increase the number of people from minority ethnic groups appointed as chairs and non-executive members of the NHS authorities and trusts and community health councillors, to reflect the composition of the population served.

5. **Service delivery**
   To provide a better service to patients by optimal use of the workforce.

6. **Doctors**
   To ensure that the time spent in higher specialist training by doctors with right of residence from minority ethnic groups equates to the time spent in higher specialist training by white doctors with right of residence.

7. **Nurses**
   NHS authorities and trusts to set a local objective to achieve equitable representation of nurses from minority ethnic backgrounds at 'G' grade (ward manager or community equivalent) within 5 years. Progress towards achieving this objective should be reviewed annually as part of the business planning cycle.

8. **Management training schemes**
   RHAs to take steps to increase each year to a locally determined level the proportion of minority ethnic people applying for and securing a place on NHS training schemes, e.g. in management, finance and other career grade training schemes. A similar requirement is placed on NHS organizations below RHA level where there are locally managed training and development schemes.

Source: Ethnic Minority Staff in the NHS: A Programme of Action (Department of Health 1993) 'less attractive' nursing specialisms such as mental health, mental handicap and geriatric nursing.

In the 1990s, attracting people from minority ethnic communities into the nursing profession has become a major problem. Akinsanya (1988), for example, notes that health visiting – which historically is accorded high status within the profession – is failing to attract nurses from minority ethnic communities. The severity of this problem is reflected in the findings of a recent Health Visitors' Association survey conducted amongst health visitors based in London. The survey, drawing on the views of 844 respondents, revealed that only 3% were from British Asian and Afro-Caribbean backgrounds (Cassidy 1995). Similarly, practice nursing – where most nurses are appointed on a 'G' grade or above – has been identified as a predominantly white specialism (Atkin & Lunt 1993).

More generally, recent statistics from the Department of Health reveal the number of applicants applying for nursing posts from minority ethnic communities is declining and that minority ethnic nurses are leaving the profession in disproportionate numbers (UNISON 1997). Table 2.2, taken from the Department of Health's annual non-medical workforce census in 1995, describes the ethnic composition of nursing, midwifery and health visiting staff.

Table 2.2 shows the NHS is finding it increasingly difficult to promote the professions of nursing, health visiting and midwifery to minority ethnic groups. This compounds the problems facing nursing bodies in attracting 'new blood' into the profession, as the NHS faces another crisis in nurse shortages across the country (Coombes 1997). The present situation is particularly worrying given that inner-city NHS trusts – those most likely to be serving multi-ethnic populations – seem to be facing the most chronic nurse shortages.

Table 2.2 Breakdown of nursing, midwifery and health visiting staff by age and ethnic group

	White	**Black**	**Asian**	**Other**	**Not stated**
All staff	88.5%	3.7%	1.2%	1.7%	4.9%
<25 years	95.2%	0.8%	1.0%	0.8%	2.3%
25–34 years	94.3%	2.2%	0.8%	2.0%	1.7%
35–44 years	91.3%	3.3%	1.6%	2.0%	1.8%
45–54 years	88.1%	5.6%	1.7%	2.9%	1.7%
55–64 years	87.3%	8.7%	1.0%	1.6%	1.5%
65+	84.0%	4.1%	0.4%	0.8%	10.7%
Unknown	0.9%	0.0%	0.0%	0.0%	99.0%

NB: Figures are based upon organizations reporting 90% or more valid ethnic codes for non-medical staff
Source: Department of Health annual non-medical workforce census (1995)

It is apparent that action at both national and local levels is required to address the shortage of minority ethnic nurses in the NHS. At a national level, as we have seen, the Department of Health's Programme of Action signals a strong commitment to the creation of a more representative nursing workforce. However, more immediate solutions to fill vacancies for nursing posts have been sought by some NHS trusts who have resorted to recruiting nurses from as far away as Finland, Canada and Australia (Porter 1996). Concern has been expressed at the appropriateness of this; it has been argued that encouraging 'blonde, blue-eyed girls' to work as nurses in this country will only create greater linguistic and cultural differences between nurse and patient, thereby reducing the quality of patient care (The Guardian 1996).

Nurse recruitment and minority ethnic groups

Little empirical research has been conducted into the reasons behind the low rates of nursing recruitment amongst minority ethnic groups. Studies conducted in the 1980s highlighted racism as a major factor deterring many potential nurses from training to become nurses (Torkington 1987, Baxter 1988a, Lee-Cunin, 1989). These studies documented how many older nurses, particularly those of Afro-Caribbean origin, felt they had been undervalued and had no hesitation in denouncing nursing, saying they would not recommend it to their children. These authors also suggested that younger members of these communities would be increasingly reluctant to expose themselves to the humiliation and degradation endured by their parents. Indeed, the Policy Studies Institute recently revealed that racial harassment was still a regular feature of the working lives of nurses, who were expected not to 'make a fuss' and to get on with their jobs. Further, management's failure to deal with racism means that racially abusive behaviour is still accepted as the norm in the nursing workplace (Beishon et al 1995).

Some writers have also highlighted cultural and religious barriers as contributing to the underrepresentation of South Asian nurses in the NHS (Rashid 1990). It has been argued by these writers that the nature of nursing work violates many of the sociocultural norms governing the behaviour of South Asian women (French et al 1994). More specifically, the physical contact between the sexes and the 'immodest' uniform worn by nurses is thought to deter many Asians from pursuing careers in nursing (Mares et al 1985). Additionally, it is felt that nursing might not be considered a 'respectable' profession amongst South Asian parents due to the low status accorded to nursing in the Indian subcontinent (Cassidy 1995, Crowe 1996, Coulling et al 1997).

However, these cultural and religious explanations for poor recruitment among minority ethnic nurses have been based more on anecdotal information than empirical research findings (Bharj 1995, Gerrish et al 1996).

Consequently, these explanations are highly questionable as they make generalizations about populations which differ enormously in terms of their cultural and religious beliefs. They also fail to consider other factors deterring students from considering a career in nursing, such as the limited efforts made by the nursing profession to attract applicants from minority ethnic groups and the lack of commitment among higher education institutions to ensure that selection procedures are fair and non-discriminatory.

EQUAL OPPORTUNITIES AND NURSE RECRUITMENT – A DEVELOPMENT PROJECT

There is clearly a need for more research to be conducted aimed at gaining clearer understanding of why nursing is failing to attract students from minority ethnic groups. This responsibility falls upon organizations concerned with nurse recruitment, such as employing bodies and educational institutions. These bodies must be willing to evaluate their own established recruitment policies and procedures to ensure that minority ethnic groups are adequately represented within their respective organizations.

At Bradford University, the School of Health Studies has recognized the severity of this recruitment problem and has taken positive steps to evaluate its own recruitment practices in a constructive way. In collaboration with local NHS trusts and funding from the West Yorkshire Education and Training Consortium, it has commissioned a two-year research and development project to investigate the low levels of recruitment and retention of South Asian workers in the health-care professions. (It is expected that the findings of this study will be available soon.)

The main aim of this study is to analyse the range of factors that contribute to the successful recruitment and retention of South Asian students into the field of professional health care. The project has three stages. First, information is being acquired through conducting indepth interviews with educational and recruitment staff within the School of Health Studies and local NHS trusts to explore their understanding of equal opportunities and their perception of the main problems in recruiting people from these groups.

Second, indepth interviews with South Asian students currently based at the School of Health Studies and local secondary schools will also be undertaken. During these interviews, students will be encouraged to express their attitudes towards health-care professions, particularly in terms of their perceptions of the nature of the work, the appropriateness of different uniforms and issues around status and the image of particular professions such as nursing. The material obtained from these interviews will be used to assess whether students experience difficulties in pursuing careers in health care and if so, to identify the nature of these difficulties.

Third, the study draws upon the views of South Asian parents of Muslim, Sikh and Hindu background to ascertain views about health care professions and assess levels of awareness and knowledge about particular careers in health care. Including parents' perspectives will provide a useful insight into prevailing cultural and religious attitudes towards different careers in health care and highlight any negative perceptions.

The study's findings will inform a protocol for better recruitment practice within the School of Health Studies. At the same time, the study will have wider implications for a range of agencies and professionals involved in promoting health care professions, ranging from professional bodies and careers officers to teachers working within local schools and colleges and recruitment staff employed by local NHS trusts. Nor are the problems facing Bradford unique and the research findings will be of value to other localities.

The few research studies which have already investigated the problem of equal opportunities in relation to nurse recruitment have highlighted the need to make greater use of the ethnic media and other non-traditional outlets as a means of promoting nursing (Bharj 1995, Turner 1996). It has also been suggested that there is a need to employ outreach workers to dispel the image of nursing as a white, middle-class profession and to actively promote nursing as a worthwhile career to members of minority ethnic groups. To this end, a number of promotional materials have already been produced in the form of booklets and videos by local professional bodies to introduce students and their families to the varied opportunities available within the nursing profession and to encourage minority ethnic groups to consider careers in nursing.

CONCLUSION

Community nursing is facing a number of challenges in its efforts to provide health care services which are responsive to the needs of multicultural populations. For nurses working in the community, there is an expectation that they will be fully capable of responding effectively to the health needs of culturally heterogeneous communities. This places a major responsibility on institutions offering nurse training to ensure that nurses are equipped with the requisite knowledge and skills to practise in multiethnic settings. Recent evidence, however, suggests the majority of nurse training institutions are only just beginning to address the adequacy of their curricula in preparing practitioners for working with multiethnic clientele (Gerrish et al 1996). It is evident that few nurse tutors accord priority to ensuring training prepares nurses to work in multiracial and multicultural settings, especially in institutions which are located in areas with small minority ethnic populations. Moreover, one can see that underrepresentation of nurse tutors from minority ethnic backgrounds in higher education institutions contributes to the exclusion of appropriate issues from the nursing curriculum.

There is clearly a need for higher education institutions to reflect on their teaching practices to ensure their curricula are culturally relevant and take account of the needs and circumstances of Britain's minority ethnic communities. Tutors should not assume that it is sufficient to teach students about specific aspects of different ethnic groups such as naming systems, diets and 'special needs', commonly known as the cookery book approach to multiculturalism. Rather, issues of race, ethnicity and culture should be examined within a broader teaching framework which integrates equal opportunities and antiracism into the curriculum as a whole. Adopting this approach increases students' knowledge about aspects of culture and religious practices, but at the same time forces them to examine the wider structural factors determining the health experiences of minority ethnic groups, thereby forming a crucial part of their learning experience.

Once within the practice setting, nursing professionals should feel able to question organizational policies and procedures to ensure nursing care is provided in an equitable and non-discriminatory way. Working within the community as members of primary health care teams, nurses are ideally placed to assess whether the services they provide are meeting the health needs of local populations effectively (see 'Questions for Discussion' at the end of the chapter).

Through identifying service deficits in relation to disadvantaged groups, nurses can and should suggest ways of improving nursing practice to meet the needs of all sections of the communities in which they work. Evaluating practice in this way should encourage nurses working in the community to become more proactive in developing services which are not only culturally sensitive but appropriate to the needs of all client groups. On a practical level, this may mean deciding to employ resources more responsively; it may mean the introduction of innovatory health care practices or it may require investigating new methods of raising client awareness of available services. Whatever changes are required, it is quite clear that it is no longer sufficient for nurses providing health care simply to acknowledge the disadvantaged status of the minority ethnic communities they work with. Rather, nurses must now act upon their knowledge and understanding of the problems facing minority groups to develop more responsive services which take account of and address their specific health needs and concerns.

QUESTIONS FOR DISCUSSION

The following checklist may help you to evaluate your own service in terms of being culturally sensitive.

◆ Access

Who is receiving which services and by what process? Are there any possible barriers to the take-up of services?

◆ Appropriateness

What types of services are being provided? How do service providers ensure that different ethnic groups feel happy about using the service?

◆ Adequacy

Do services address the needs of all ethnic groups in the local population?

◆ Equity

Are services being provided to individuals from different ethnic groups in a fair and equitable manner?

ANNOTATED BIBLIOGRAPHY

Ahmad W I U 1993 'Race' and health in contemporary Britain. Open University Press, Buckingham

This useful introductory text brings together writings on health policy, research and practice within the context of wider political, economic and institutional structures and the ideology of racism. The book reviews and advances health-care provision and delivery in relation to minority ethnic populations, focusing on issues of particular concern to community nurses such as mental health and elderly care.

Bowler I 1993 'They're not the same as us': midwives' stereotypes of South Asian descent maternity patients. Sociology of Health And Illness 15 (2)

Bowler's ethnographic study of maternity care and South Asian patients serves as a useful example of the way in which stereotypes are used by health professionals to perpetuate inequalities in service delivery. What makes this article particularly readable is the way in which Bowler manages to highlight common attitudes and perceptions of midwives towards the patients in her study and contextualize them within the wider literature on patient typification.

Gerrish K, Husband C, Mackenzie J 1996 Nursing for a multi-ethnic society. Open University Press, Buckingham

This book reports the findings of a two-year research project which was funded by the English National Board of Nursing, Midwifery and Health Visiting to examine the extent to which nurses and midwives are prepared to meet the

health-care needs of minority ethnic communities. Focusing specifically on preregistration programmes, the authors provide a wide-ranging and critical overview of educational curricula and approaches presently on offer to student nurses and midwives to enable them to meet the health needs of ethnically diverse populations.

Beishon S, Virdee S, Hagell A 1995 Nursing in a multi-ethnic NHS. Policy Studies Institute, London

This book looks at the experiences of nurses and midwives this time in relation to equal opportunities and employment within the NHS. It draws upon data collected from both a qualitative study of six nurse employers and 150 interviews and a large-scale postal survey of 14 000 staff. The authors provide evidence to suggest the continued existence of racial harassment and unfair promotion procedures within many workplaces which leads them to the conclusion that there are still significant gaps between equal opportunities policy and practice within the NHS.

REFERENCES

Agbolegbe R 1984 Fighting the racist. Nursing Times 80 (16): 18–20
Ahmad W I U 1996a Family obligations and social change among Asian communities. In: Ahmad W I U, Atkin K (eds) Race and community care. Open University Press, Buckingham
Ahmad W I U 1996b The trouble with culture. In: Kelleher D, Hillier S (eds) Researching cultural differences in health. Routledge, London
Akinsanya J 1988 Ethnic minority nurses, midwives and health visitors: what role for them in the National Health Service? New Community 14 (3): 444–450
Anionwu E 1993 Sickle cell and thalassaemia: community experiences and official response. In: Ahmad W I U (eds) Race and health in contemporary Britain. Open University Press, Buckingham
Atkin K, Lunt N 1993 Nurses count: a national census of practice nurses. Social Policy Research Unit, York
Atkin K, Rollings J 1993 Community care in a multi-racial Britain. HMSO, London
Atkin K, Badger F, Cameron E, Evers H 1989 Black elders knowledge and future use of community services. New Community 15 (5): 439–446
Badger F, Cameron E, Evers H 1990 Slipping through the net. Health Service Journal 100 (5184): 86–87
Balarajan R, Bulosu L 1990 Mortality among immigrants in England and Wales. In: Britton M (ed) Mortality and geography: a review of the mid 1980s. OPCS, London
Balarajan R, Raleigh V 1995 Ethnicity and health in England. HMSO, London
Baxter C 1988a The black nurse: an endangered species. National Extension College, London
Baxter C 1988b Culture shock. Nursing Times 84 (2): 36–36
Baxter C 1997 The case for bilingual workers within the maternity services. British Journal of Midwifery 5 (9): 568–572
Beech B 1991 Who's holding your baby? Bedford Square Press, London
Beishon S, Virdee S, Hagell A 1995 Nursing in a multi-ethnic NHS. Policy Studies Institute, London
Beliappa J 1991 Illness or distress? Alternative models of mental health. Confederation of Indian Organisations, London
Bharj K K 1995 Nurse recruitment: an Asian response. Race Relations Research Unit, Bradford
Blakemore K, Boneham M 1994 Age, race and ethnicity: a comparative approach. Open University Press, Buckingham
Bowler I 1993a 'They're not the same as us': midwives' stereotypes of South Asian descent maternity patients. Sociology of Health and Illness 15 (2): 157–178

Bowler I 1993b Stereotypes of women of Asian descent in midwifery: some evidence. Midwifery 9: 7–16

Butt J, Mirza K 1996 Social care and black communities. Race Equality Unit, London

Cartwright A 1979 The dignity of labour? Tavistock, London

Cassidy 1995 Ethnic dilemma. Nursing Times 91 (42): p 18

Chevannes M 1991 Access to health care for black people. Health Visitor 64 (1): 16–17

Colman D, Salt J 1995 Ethnicity in the 1991 Census Vol 1: demographic characteristics of the ethnic minority population. HMSO, London

Combes G, Schonueld A 1992 Life will never be the same again. Health Education Authority, London

Commission for Racial Equality 1987 Ethnic origins of nurses applying for and in training – a survey. CRE, London

Coombes R 1997 NHS overlooks black recruits as seniors bale out. Nursing Times 93 (93): p 7

Coulling et al 1997 Plain tales from the Punjab. Nursing Times 93 (14): 30–33

Crowe M 1996 Cancer nursing in Pakistan. Journal of Cancer Care 5 (4): 179–181

Department of Health 1991 The patient's charter. HMSO, London

Department of Health 1992 The health of the nation: a strategy for health in England. HMSO, London

Department of Health 1993a Ethnic minority staff in the NHS: a programme of action. NHS Management Executive, London

Department of Health 1993b Maternity service for Asian women. NHS Management Executive, London

Donovan J L 1984 Ethnicity and disease: a research review. Social Science and Medicine 19 (7): 663–670

Doyal L, Hunt G, Mello J 1981 Your life in their hands: migrant workers in the National Health Service. Report of a preliminary survey. Polytechnic of North London, Social Science Research Council, London

Faden R 1991 Autonomy, choice, and the new reproductive technologies: the role of informed consent in prenatal genetic diagnosis. In: Rodin J, Collins A (eds) Women and new reproductive technologies: medical, psychological, legal and ethical dilemmas. Hillsdale, New York

Foster M 1988 Health visitors' perspectives on working in a multi-ethnic society: Health Visitor 61: 275–278

French S, Watters D, Matthews D 1994 Nursing as a career choice for women in Pakistan. Journal Of Advanced Nursing 19 (3): 140–151

Gerrish K, Husband C, Mackenzie J 1996 Nursing for a multi-ethnic society. Open University Press, Buckingham

Greater London Action for Race Equality (GLARE) 1987 No alibi, no excuse. A progress report on the development of equal opportunities in employment in London's health authorities. GLARE, London

Guardian 1996 Boost to nurse recruitment as MP apologises. 29.11.96

Health Education Authority (HEA) 1994 Health-related resources for black and minority ethnic groups. HEA, London

King Edward's Hospital Fund for London 1990 Racial equality: the nursing profession. Equal opportunities task force occasional paper no. 6. King's Fund Publishing Office, London

Koch H 1994 Towards total quality in community nursing services. Longman, Harlow

Larbie J 1985 Black women and the maternity services. National Extension College Health Education Council, London

Lee-Cunin M 1989 Daughters of Seacole. West Yorkshire Low Pay Unit, Batley

Leeds Family Health Services Authority (LFHSA) 1992 Research into the uptake of maternity services as provided by primary health care teams to women from black and ethnic minorities. LFHSA, Leeds

Mares P, Henley A, Baxter C 1985 Healthcare in multiracial Britain. National Extension College/Health Education Council, Cambridge

Marmot A, Adelstein A, Bulusu L 1984 Immigrant mortality in England and Wales: 1970–1978. HMSO, London

Murphy K, Clark J M 1993 Nurses' experience of caring for ethnic minority clients. Journal of Advanced Nursing 18: 442–450

National Association Of Health Authorities (NAHA) 1988 Action not words – a strategy to improve health services for black and minority ethnic groups. NAHA, Birmingham

Nazroo J 1997 The health of Britain's ethnic minorities. Policy Studies Institute, London

Parkside Community Health Council (PCHC) 1992 Women speak out. Parkside CHC, London

Pearson M 1985 Racial equality and good practice in maternity care. National Extension College/Health Education Council, London

Pearson M 1987 Racism: the great divide. Nursing Times 83 (24): 24–26

Phoenix A 1990 Black women and the maternity services. In: Garcia J, Kilpatrick R, Richards M (eds) The politics of maternity care. Oxford University Press, New York

Porter R 1996 Poor start on the Finnish line. Nursing Times 92 (50): 20–21

Rashid 1990 Asian doctors and nurses in the NHS. In: Mcavoy B, Donaldson L (eds) Health care for Asians. Oxford University Press, Oxford

Rocheron Y 1988 The Asian mother and baby campaign: the construction of ethnic minorities health needs. Critical Social Policy 22: 4–23

Rudat K 1994 Black and minority ethnic groups in England. Health Education Authority, London

Shackman J 1984 The right to be understood – a handbook on working with, employing and training community interpreters. Health Education Authority, London

Shah R 1992 The silent minority: children with disabilities in Asian families. National Children's Bureau, London

Torkington P 1984 Blaming black women – rickets and racism. In: O'Sullivan S (ed) Women's health: a spare rib reader. Pandora, London

Torkington P 1987 Sorry wrong colour. Nursing Times 83 (24): 27–28

Torkington P 1991 Black health: a political issue. Catholic Association for Racial Justice/Liverpool Institute for Higher Education, London

Townsend P, Davison N 1982 Inequalities in health: the Black report. Penguin, Harmondsworth

Turner J 1995 Towards a fair admissions policy? Leeds College of Health, Leeds

UKCC 1992 Code of professional conduct. United Kingdom Central Council for Nursing, Midwifery and Health Visiting, London

Ullah S 1994 The health needs of Bangladeshi women for maternity care. Bradford Family Health Services Authority, Bradford

UNISON 1997 Black women's employment and pay. UNISON, London

Walker R, Ahmad W I U 1994 Asian and black elders and community care: a survey of care providers. New Community 20 (4): 635–646

Watters C 1996 Representations and realities: black people, community care and mental illness. In: Ahmad W I U, Atkin K (eds) Race and community care. Open University Press, Buckingham

Williams 1989 Social policy: a critical introduction. Polity Press, Cambridge

Woollett A, Dosanjh-Matwala N 1990a Pregnancy and antenatal care: the attitudes and experiences of Asian women. Child Care, Health and Development 16 (1): 63–78

Woollett A, Dosanjh-Matwala N 1990b Postnatal care: the attitudes and experiences of Asian women in East London. Midwifery 6: 178–184

3

Skill mix in primary care – shifting the balance

Susan Jenkins-Clarke

KEY ISSUES

- ◆ Issues of skill mix are vital in the development of community nursing.
- ◆ There is no consensus regarding the different definitions of skill mix in primary health care teams.
- ◆ Factors important in skill mix enquiries include current workload, delegation and attitudes to delegation.

INTRODUCTION

This chapter explores skill mix in primary care. Many issues surround this concept although some of these, such as delegation, are concepts in their own right. However, they also need to be recognized as an integral part of skill mix. The chapter demonstrates how the background and current context of primary care delivery today have shaped how we measure skill mix.

An enquiry, undertaken by the University of York, was commissioned by the Department of Health in response to anxieties expressed about recruitment and retention into general practice. Although the central focus of this enquiry was the general practitioner, the study could not ignore the contribution of community nurses in the delivery of primary care.

The results of the study, outlined in this chapter, are based on detailed data collected from all members of primary health care teams (PHCTs) working in 10 general practices across the Midlands and the North of England. These data related to workload, current referral and potential delegation. Data relating to teamworking, patients' views about the accessibility of members of PHCTs and shared care management of patients with chronic diseases are reported elsewhere (Jenkins-Clarke et al 1997). Before specifically discussing skill mix and outlining the study's results, a brief introduction to the current changes in primary health care is necessary.

In the National Health Service (NHS) and in the primary care sector in particular, the balance between care providers is of utmost importance in ensuring that good quality, cost-effective care can be delivered to patients and clients, both in their own homes and in general practice surgeries. Care delivered to patients in the acute and primary care sectors has undergone rapid change largely due to the creation of the internal market and, in the primary care sector, with the advent of general practice fundholding and locality commissioning. These changes have led to a shift in the balance of power from hospitals to the community and the emergence of a primary care-led NHS. For the purposes of this chapter, we focus our attention on three background issues important in primary care today: workforce themes; boundary definitions and enhanced roles; and changes in workload.

Workforce themes

With the medical and nursing workforces currently undergoing change, recruitment and retention are reaching almost crisis proportions, particularly amongst GPs. In particular, there is a fall in the number of doctors being attracted into general practice and undergoing vocational training (Handysides 1994), a reduction in the number of training posts on offer and a rise in the number of general practitioners taking early retirement (McBride & Metcalfe 1995). There has also been a rise in the number of part-time doctors (Department of Health 1995) and, in particular, part-time female general practitioners (Leigh 1996).

Within the nursing workforce, and in contrast to the above, the numbers of practice nurses have trebled since the late 1980s (Atkin & Lunt 1993). This rapid growth has generated concerns about working conditions and education and training. There has been a fall in health visitor recruitment, however, over the same period and little change in the numbers of district nurses (Department of Health 1994).

Boundary definitions and enhanced roles

The emergence of new professional groups is also taking place in response, at least in part, to the changing requirements of primary care delivery. For example, nurse practitioner courses are gaining in popularity, as are clinical nurse specialists. As well as the emergence of new professional groups within nursing itself, there are also increasing numbers of health-care assistants being trained and employed to work alongside nursing members of PHCTs.

Currently practice nursing is the main focus for enhanced roles in health care. The advent of mandatory health checks for people over the age of 75 and the screening, immunization and vaccination targets set out in the Health of the Nation report (1992) has resulted in expanded roles for practice nurses. Other examples of enhanced roles being undertaken by practice nurses relate to the treatment of minor illnesses; Marsh & Dawes (1995) reported that practice nurses could deal with 86% of minor illness consultations without referring back to the doctor. Practice nurses are also increasingly taking part in chronic disease management, with particular reference to asthma (Charlton et al 1991), diabetes (Carr et al 1991) and hypertension (Jewell & Hope 1988).

Looking to the future, the triage function of nurses in primary care is gaining popularity. With the advent of telephone triage and nurse prescribing this trend will probably be extended – possibly to other groups of nurses and with an extended formulary. These are just two examples of nurses adapting and taking the opportunity to create new roles in the ever-changing context of primary-care delivery. The policy focus with regards to enhanced roles highlights the increasing popularity and demand for nurse or health-care practitioners. The concept of nurse practitioners developed over two decades ago in the USA and Canada and it was widely reported that this group of nurses could provide safe and effective care (Spitzer et al 1974, Denton et al 1983). In 1986 Baroness Cumberlege recommended the introduction of the nurse practitioner into primary care in the UK. The controversy surrounding the role of the nurse practitioner lies in whether these specialist nurses substitute for doctors or whether they fulfil a complementary role, as favoured by commentators such as Stilwell et al (1987) and Salisbury & Tettersall (1988).

Changes in workload

All community nurses report an increase in workload, attributable in general terms to government legislation such as the Community Care Act (Department of Health 1990) and the Health of the Nation (Department of Health 1992). As outlined in Chapter 1, the resulting shift from secondary to primary care means that more people are being cared for in their own homes, patients are discharged early from hospital and there has been a move to shared care in the management of chronic disease such as asthma and diabetes. These factors, coupled with an increasingly ageing population, all contribute to increased workload for community nurses.

Seccombe et al (1994) report that nearly two-thirds (65%) of community nurses recorded working extra hours – in contrast to their hospital colleagues where 54% reported working excess hours. Both district nurses and health visitors report a trend of longer working hours since 1990. Health visitors are likely to work more hours than district nurses – an average of 9.4 h per week compared to district nurses reporting 7.5 h per week. Such increases carry with them a lowering of job satisfaction for the nursing workforce (Wade 1993).

UNDERSTANDING SKILL MIX

The goal of good quality, cost-effective care in general practice remains a central objective of primary care changes. Thus, the balance between members of staff is crucial and it is this concept of balance which lies at the centre of skill mix amongst PHCTs. The skill mix of a team can, in principle, be measured in a number of ways:

◆ in terms of disciplines;
◆ levels of qualifications within a discipline or relevant experience;
◆ competence/skills.

Given the mixture of professional groups in PHCTs, it is probably inappropriate to use team members' qualifications or experience as a direct measure for aggregating across the PHCT. It would, however, be appropriate to make an assessment of the mixture of GP qualifications in a PHCT or the mixture of nurses within a PHCT, in terms of both experience and qualifications.

There have been a number of skill mix studies within nursing which have reported fundamentally differing conclusions. On one hand, some studies support the notion of a rich skill mix (i.e. more qualified nurses) while others support the opposite view – increasing the numbers of unqualified staff. Interestingly, the studies supporting a richer skill mix relate skill mixing to the delivery of good quality care (Carr-Hill et al 1992, Bagust et al 1992) in contrast to the latter view (such as The Value for Money Unit's report, 1992) – one explanation possibly being the focus on the narrow field of task analysis. McKenna's (1995) comprehensive review of skill mix amongst nurses in the acute sector explores the relationship between rich and weak skill mixes and the quality of care delivered. In primary care, there is a need to extend such enquiry to an interprofessional level and to examine the relationships between medical, nursing and paramedical staff.

Although skill mix could potentially be measured in any of the ways mentioned, such an approach would only partly capture the concept of skill mix. Clues to the elusive nature of the concept lie in the dynamics of PHCTs, how these teams function and the extent to which workload is, or could be, shared amongst teams. Consequently a description of working patterns and current workload of members of PHCTs is a useful way of beginning to understand skill mix.

Given the acknowledged increase in workload, measuring workload activity and working patterns serves to highlight the issue of workload management, the possibility of redistributing workload amongst members of the PHCT and the identification of referral pathways. Realistically, the focal point of workload shift is whether any activities currently carried out by the general practitioner can be appropriately and acceptably delegated to other members of the team. The possibility of redistributing workload in PHCTs raises the need for baseline data on the work patterns of the doctors and nurses working in PHCTs; the extent of referral between members of the team; and the acceptability and appropriateness of delegation from the GP to other members of the PHCT.

The study reported here addresses these issues. Data were collected across 10 sites from all members of the PHCT using a variety of instruments. Information was collected about doctors' and community nurses' workload; about whether there was any possibility of workload being delegated/referred to other people; and what the teams' views were about this. The broad aim of this enquiry was to propose ways of examining the constraints upon, and the opportunities for, spreading workload more effectively and efficiently amongst members of the PHCT. Prior to addressing these questions, definitions of the two concepts of skill mix and PHCTs require exploration.

Towards defining skill mix

An essential first step in any research enquiry is to define one's subject matter. So, what do we mean by skill mix? It is an elusive concept and therefore difficult to define in terms of the delivery of health care; there are, however, numerous examples of definitions of skill mix in other fields, including occupational sociology and industrial sociology. One of the definitions most relevant to the NHS workforce is that of the Health Policy and Economic Research Unit at the British Medical Association:

> *The balance between trained and untrained, qualified and unqualified and supervisory and operative staff within a service area as well as between different groups.* (Nessling 1990)

It is the notion of balance in the above definition which is central to the concept of skill mixing in general practice and which implies flexibility – a concept at the heart of recent White Papers on primary care from both Conservative and Labour governments.

Towards defining the primary health care team

Unlike the definition of skill mix referred to above, defining what we mean by primary health care teams is less difficult. But although PHCTs are familiar terrain for community nurses, opinions vary as to the precise membership of such teams. However, there appears to be a consensus that there is a 'core' team, comprising GPs, practice nurses, district nurses, health visitors, a practice manager and clerical staff. Sometimes other professional groups are included, sometimes excluded. As an illustration, in the 10 practices participating in the York study, the configuration of PHCTs was as shown in Figure 3.1.

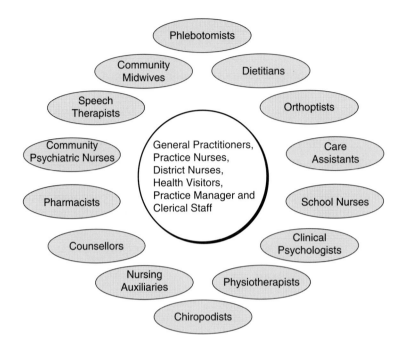

Fig. 3.1 Composition of primary health-care teams.

Delegation

The terms 'delegation' and 'referral' are used interchangeably throughout this chapter. The potential for substitution depends on the current division of labour and the size of the market; typically, in the UK, general practices are relatively small 'firms' so that 'substitution' may actually involve employing additional staff. Empirical examinations of skill mix in the health services have usually been concerned with larger groups of staff and/or staff belonging to one professional group only – for example, nurses on a ward. Thus, while a broad-brush or macro examination might show, for example, that 20% of a doctor's time could be substituted by a mix of practice manager and practice nurse time (and perhaps other members of the PHCT), the practicalities of weaving together such a collection of part-time workers into a coherent team may be insurmountable.

The possible pitfalls of shifting workload from the GP to other members of the team should also be addressed. There may be fragmentation of care and/or loss of 'whole-person' holistic care, both of which may reduce the quality of care. Moreover, there are no systematic research data on such a shift. Interviews with patients or self-completion questionnaires typically refer to the anticipated or previous consultation. Often they ask questions such as, 'Do you want to see a particular GP/nurse?', 'Were you able to see the GP/

nurse you wanted to?', 'How long did you have to wait?'. Such questions relate to the instantaneous relationship which might be, or was, established during the 10-minute interaction, as opposed to any assessment of satisfaction with the current encounter in terms of the quality of a relationship previously established.

Delegation of workload and particularly transferring workload from doctor to nurse (or to any other members of the team) mean that GPs may change the balance of their own activities, possibly towards more intensive management of more 'serious' problems. Moreover, practices with many non-medical clinicians may be able to deal more comprehensively with a wider range of work, thereby increasing the range and quality of services provided. This could include dealing with problems that would otherwise be referred elsewhere for treatment. More prosaically, it may simply ensure that the current level of activity in primary care can be maintained and possibly increased (Jenkins-Clarke & Carr-Hill 1996).

There are a number of examples of delegation in the literature, the majority devoted to delegation from doctor to nurse. According to Robinson (1990), this is because many of the examples of increased workload fall within the scope of nurses. Marsh & Davies (1995) describe a somewhat extreme scenario – of GPs delegating to other members of the PHCT – that would result in GPs' lists doubling in size. A pilot study reported by the Georgian Society (1991) found that GPs responded positively to the extension of the role of the practice nurse in providing counselling and advice and patients having direct access to them but they had reservations about the evolution of that role, particularly towards independent nursing diagnosis and initiation of treatment. This was subsequently confirmed by Atkin & Lunt (1995). In their national sample, Robinson et al (1993) found that 93% of GPs would welcome the expansion of the work undertaken by practice nurses and nearly a third of them (30%) wished to see this group of nurses acting as independent practitioners (Table 3.1).

Whilst the main focus of delegation describes the referral pathways between doctor and nurse, there are examples of skill mixing between nurses themselves, usually in the form of delegation from highly qualified nurses to those less qualified. The Value for Money Report (1992) concluded that the number of qualified nurses could be halved if tasks were delegated to less qualified staff. This study evoked considerable criticism, mainly because district nursing was regarded as being more than a series of practical activities. This PCHT role encompasses 'core activities' such as assessment, monitoring of standards, teaching and evaluating care delivery.

The advent of GP fundholding has brought these issues to the fore and community nursing services, alongside their GP colleagues, need to address concerns about the delivery of 'appropriate' nursing care using personnel

Table 3.1 Tasks that GPs expected practice nurses to undertake

Task	% of GPs expecting practice nurses to undertake task (n = 1748–1797)
Measuring blood pressure	99.2
Sterilizing and maintaining equipment	95.5
Running health promotion clinics	92.7
Advising on and giving travel immunization	92.4
Carrying out venepuncture for blood sampling	89.5
Measuring blood glucose level	85.5
Performing cervical smears	84.1
Performing childhood immunization	82.1
Helping minor surgery clinics	76.0
Measuring peak expiratory flow rate	75.4
Examining for breast lumps	64.5
Performing electrocardiograph recording	61.1
Carrying out home visiting of over 75-year-olds	55.2
Recognizing anxiety and depression	53.6
Observing skin for signs of disease	38.4
Carrying out home visits for other reasons	32.4
Making referrals directly to social services	31.1
Summarizing medical notes	27.5
Performing stethoscopic examination of heart/chest	8.2
Making referrals directly to hospital departments	7.0

n = range of number of respondents replying to questions
Source: Robinson et al 1993

with the appropriate skills to deliver such care safely, efficiently and effectively.

The new GP contract (Department of Health 1990) saw attitudes towards delegation shift. Prior to the new contract, GPs were far more cautious in their consideration of transferring activities to other members of staff. According to Bowling (1981), the reasons for this were that doctors feared loss of independence, more work being created and the loss of the doctor–patient relationship. These fears remain today but are now set against a background of extended nurse roles in areas such as shared care of chronic disease management, screening and the diagnosis and treatment of minor illness. Fragmentation of care is frequently voiced as the downside of delegation, conflicting with the ethos of the delivery of holistic care.

The picture, then, is a divergent one, with advocates for referring many more activities on to members of PHCTs on the one hand and on the other, those who fear that such fragmentation of care can only lead to weaker doctor–patient relationships (Lloyd 1994). There is no doubt, however, that the past decade has seen the expansion of PHCTs and that as these teams expand, so will the *modus operandi* of the individuals working in the team.

Against this background, the Department of Health commissioned a study undertaken by the Centre for Health Economics entitled 'The Interface between the Doctor and Other Members of the Primary Health Care Team'. The remainder of this chapter summarizes this study with a discussion of the issues arising from the findings and the way ahead.

THE STUDY

This study was commissioned in response to growing concerns about the labour force crisis in general practice and the effect of this upon the workload of general practitioners and community nurses.

Ten practices were invited to take part; these were 'ordinary' practices from five family health service authorities (FHSAs) and were regarded as 'typical' rather than 'leading edge' practices. Some were teaching practices, some were fundholders (six) and all were equally divided between rural and urban settings. The criteria for choice were: ratio of practice nurses: GPs; three or more GP partners per practice; and the presence of a practice manager.

Data were collected from GPs, practice nurses (PNs), district nurses (DNs), health visitors (HVs) and midwives as well as practice managers, administrative staff and patients (those attending surgery during the 2-week observation period and patients registered as asthmatics and diabetics in practice registers). The type of data collected is shown in Figure 3.2.

Data were collected as follows.

◆ 836 consultations were observed by research nurses.
◆ 51 GPs completed workload (DDRB) diaries and delegation diaries.
◆ 77 nurses completed workload and delegation diaries.
◆ 2000 patients completed questionnaires on their general attitudes to the practice.
◆ For each practice, data on structure and management of the practice were collected.
◆ Basic demographic data and views about teamworking were ascertained for each of the professional team members (n = 208).
◆ For asthmatics (n = 1100) and diabetics (n = 280), information was extracted from medical records to accompany responses to self-completed postal questionnaires.
◆ Qualitative data were obtained from focus group discussions in each of the 10 participating practices.
◆ These data were collected over a 2-week observation period in each participating practice.

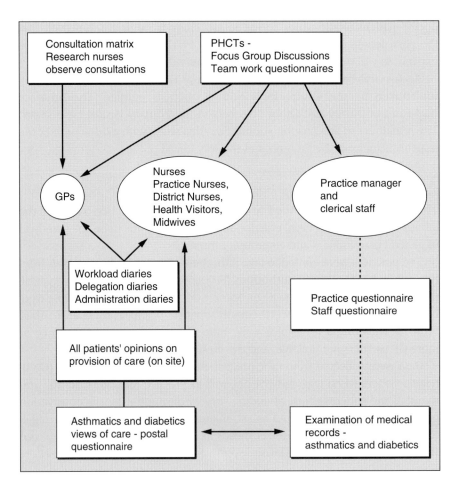

Fig. 3.2 The flow of data instruments.

The findings and discussion reported here are based on four instruments used in the study. First, workload diaries were completed by community nurses over a 2-week period at each site. Nurses were asked to complete activity diaries for the entire week to include activities on and off surgery premises (such as home visits), distinguishing between treatment, immunization, diagnostic testing, screening, health education (to patients and clients, either singly or in groups), hygiene, advice and reassurance, teaching, discussion and paperwork. Diary entries were required for each 30-min period of the working day. The results presented here focus on those completed by practice nurses (28), district nurses (30) and health visitors (13). In total there were 323 diary sheets completed by these three groups, representing 3239 diary entries.

The second instrument used to generate findings relating to delegation was created by research nurses observing GP consultations, recording the content of the consultation and assigning the process and outcome of these activities every 30 s under a series of headings. In total, research nurses sat in on 836 consultations divided between morning and afternoon/evening surgeries. Potential opportunities for delegation were identified at this point, in discussion with the GP being observed.

Third, a delegation diary was completed by practice nurses, district nurses and GPs during the second week of data collection at each site.

The fourth instrument was that of the focus group discussion; these were held on two occasions at each site – prior to the start of data collection and then again at the end of the 2-week observation period. All members of the PHCT were invited to attend these discussion groups.

The results presented here focus on workload and delegation. In particular, we address three objectives of the study.

◆ Objective 1   *To document the current pattern of activities and interactions between the GP and other members of the PHCT.*
◆ Objective 2   *To assess the potential for some of the GP's activities to be performed by other members of the team in terms of the mix of skills required.*
◆ Objective 3   *To examine the attitudes of GPs towards delegation, of the practice managers and nurses to taking on other responsibilities and everyone's attitudes to team management.*

Workload

Workload diaries completed by doctors and community nurses were used to address objective one. Using the nurses' workload diaries (n = 71), with diary entries recording the previous 30 minutes' activities – we found that

◆ For practice nurses, the four main categories in order of activity were diagnostic testing, followed by discussion and paperwork, treatment and health education. There may be some overlap between the activities of treatment and diagnostic testing, but with regards to health education and discussion and paperwork, about an eighth of the activities recorded by practice nurses involved the former and about a fifth of time was spent on the latter.
◆ For district nurses, the four main categories in order of activity were treatment, discussion and paperwork, advice and reassurance and hygiene. This group of nurses thus spent about a third of their time on activities involving treatment and over a quarter of their time on activities involving paperwork and discussion. Only district nurses recorded the activity of teaching, spending 2% of their time on this activity, defined as teaching professional groups (i.e. trainee/student health professionals) as distinct from patient or client teaching which was recorded elsewhere.
◆ For health visitors, the four main categories in order of activity were

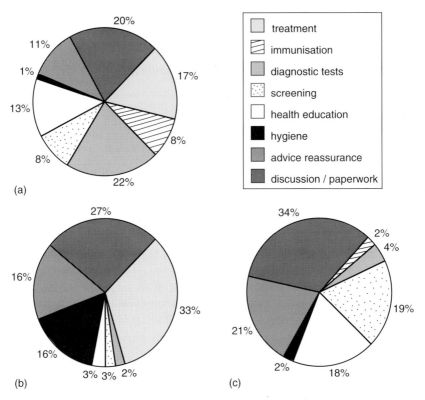

Fig. 3.3 Patterns of activity by: (a) practice nurses, (b) district nurses (excluding teaching at 2%), (c) health visitors.

discussion and paperwork, advice and reassurance, screening and health education. Health visitors record more 'focused' activities than either of the other two groups, particularly as there may be some overlap between the two categories of advice and health education (Fig. 3.3).

Delegation

To address objective two, observation techniques were employed with data being recorded by research nurses sitting in on GP consultations at each of the 10 sites. Usually, a morning and an afternoon/evening surgery per GP were observed, recording the content of the consultation every 30 s onto a matrix. At the end of each consultation, the research nurse confirmed the activity taking place in that consultation with the GP and also asked him/her whether there was any activity in that particular consultation which could have been passed onto someone else.

It is clear from Table 3.2 that there is a wide variation between the 10 practices as to the willingness to delegate – a minimum amount of delegation being identified in practice 4 (14%) with over three times as much being

Table 3.2 Percentage of consultations observed by research nurses when GPs agreed there was a delegatable element

Practice	No. of consults	Percentage of consultations			
		With potential for referral			Capable of being referred in their entirety
		To any source	To current team	To enhanced team	
1	89	44.9	19.1	22.5	21.4
2	81	50.6	34.6	18.5	17.3
3	72	52.8	34.7	25.0	27.8
4	93	23.7	14.0	15.1	6.4
5	76	56.6	43.4	14.5	23.7
6	92	34.8	27.2	13.0	8.7
7	125	28.0	18.4	12.0	20.8
8	55	49.1	45.5	9.1	18.2
9	85	31.8	25.9	7.1	17.7
10	68	30.9	20.6	13.2	7.4
All	836	39.0	26.9	15.0	17.3

There were also 141 consultations (17%) where the GP claimed that **all** of the consultation could have been delegated

When the GPs agreed there was a potential for referral, they were then asked whether that was to a member of the current PHCT or to a professional who could in principle be part of a PHCT but was not currently part of their team

identified in practice 8 (46%). In this latter practice nearly half of all consultations contained at least one activity with a potential for delegation. A similar range of consultations is found amongst sites where GPs could see the potential to delegate to an 'enhanced team'.

The totals reveal that two-thirds of the potential for delegation was reported to be to members of the existing PHCT and about one-third to members of an 'enhanced team'. In the case of the latter, respondents were asked to record, in their own words, the professional groups who might make up the membership of an 'enhanced team' – in other words a form of 'wish list'.

It is also worth noting the last column of Table 3.2 which shows that 17% of all consultations, according to the GP, could have been delegated in their entirety – 141 consultations in total. The members of staff to whom GPs were most likely to delegate were, in the current team, practice nurses and, in the enhanced team, nurse practitioners.

What were GPs prepared to delegate?

There were 269 opportunities for delegation identified to the current team and 150 opportunities for delegation to an enhanced team. Ranking these

Table 3.3 Opportunities to delegate from observed consultations (using the consultation matrices)

	Potentially delegatable to current team (%)	Potentially delegatable to enhanced team (%)
Skin complaints	12.4	12.1
Screening	16.4	5.2
Contraception	8.4	14.7
Prescribing	12.2	6.9
Advice and reassurance	21.6	25.9
Base N for all	269	150

opportunities for the current team, nearly a quarter refer to advice and reassurance, followed by screening, treatment of skin complaints and prescribing. To an enhanced team, once more advice and reassurance is the most common followed again by treatment of skin complaints and contraception (defined as pill checks, interuterine device checks and hormone replacement therapy checks).

Attitudes

Focus group discussions (FGDs) were used to address objective three. All members of the PHCT (however defined) were invited to attend these discussions. One was held at the beginning of the data collection at the start of the first week and the second held at the end of the site visit. The same themes were scheduled for discussion at both meetings and these discussions yielded rich qualitative data about members' views on teamworking, roles and boundaries and feelings about delegating workload to each other.

These 20 FGDs revealed that members of the teams had reservations about delegation, with particular reference to the complexity of the consultation itself. In summary, these reservations were: the complexity of consultations; willingness of patients to see other members of the team; and the impact of delegation on other team members.

The first reservation – that of complexity – was universally acknowledged across all practices and raised a number of subsidiary issues relating to splitting up the consultation via processes such as triage. For example, questions such as who is the 'best' person to undertake this role and what might be the education and training consequences of such a development are issues which require further investigation.

The second reservation – that of patients' willingness to see other members of the PHCT – was in fact addressed in this study. Nearly 2000 patients were asked a variety of questions relating to the accessibility of members of the team. About two-thirds said they preferred continuity. However, half said that they would have preferred to see another doctor if they could have seen one sooner than their own or would have preferred to see a nurse rather than any GP if they could see her/him sooner than another doctor.

Regarding the impact that delegation might have on other team members, discussions on this topic often led to a discussion of roles and boundaries of community nurses. Enhanced roles or the extension of nurse roles were frequently referred to, usually regarding the extension of the practice nurse role into areas such as diagnosing minor self-limiting illnesses and the ability to prescribe. Whilst many nurses felt that this would be a positive step forward, there were some differences of opinion as to the desirability of such a move. Some nurses felt strongly that they did not have the necessary training to undertake these roles, whilst others felt that, with suitable and appropriate training, they would welcome the opportunity to expand their roles.

The role of the nurse practitioner featured in these discussions and also in the surgery observation sessions when GPs discussed with research nurses the various activities thought to be amenable to potential delegation. There was considerable confusion amongst members of the PHCT as to the role of nurse practitioners; GPs assumed that nurse practitioners were able to prescribe and indeed saw this activity as being the 'flagship' of this extended role and that nurses would be able to prescribe from an extensive range of drugs and not be limited by the current formulary for nurse prescribing. This confusion was apparent in the following GP quote:

> *I wouldn't perceive them (nurse practitioners) to have particularly different skills to the practice nurse ... extended a bit perhaps. I would find it frustrating to wait for a doctor to write a prescription for an antibiotic. They clearly know how to manage the problem; they've written the script out for you and they're waiting for you to put an illegible scribble at the bottom ... that must be quite irritating ... waiting for a doctor to come and say that's a cellulitis ... something they know perfectly well.*

PRIMARY CARE SKILL MIX – AN AGENDA FOR SCRUTINY

The subtitle of this chapter is 'shifting the balance' – a notion integral to the definition of skill mix. It is this concept of balance which is crucial to skill mix exercises and central to many of the recent primary-care developments. The concepts of integrated care, shared care, care pathways and care management, for example, represent examples of primary care which have, at their centres, this notion of balance. The study outlined here provides evidence of the potential for shifting workload around amongst members of PHCTs. Moreover, it is seen as acceptable, both amongst those providing and those receiving care. The study shows an essential first step is to assess current workload activity before proceeding to discussions as to how this workload can be transferred to other members of the team.

Workload assessment – the first step

The literature indicates that both doctors and nurses have experienced an increase in workload, particularly since the introduction of GP fundholding and the shift from acute to community care. GPs mainly cite an increase in administrative tasks as increased workload whereas practice nurse workload indicates an increase in the scope and content of their practice (Atkin & Lunt 1995). These authors maintain that because the scope and content of practice nurse workload are changing and since this group of nurses appears to be taking on most of this work, this guarantees the future of practice nurses. It is this scenario which has fuelled the debate on workload management.

In our study, we found that, according to their own reports, individual nurses concentrate on different aspects of their job description. However, in general, a practice nurse does appear to be spending more time on diagnosis than either of the other two groups of community nurses, a district nurse more time on treatment than other groups and a health visitor more time on screening than either of the other two groups.

Discussion and paperwork have a high profile in all community nurses' activities, particularly so for district nurses and health visitors. This may be a reflection of their 'attached' status and the necessity of recording workload and other information for health authority purposes. For health visitors, the amount of time spent on discussion and paperwork may be accounted for by participation in case conferences and other multiagency working.

Slightly surprising is the finding that health visitors report spending only a sixth of their time on health education activities whilst practice nurses spend over an eighth (although health visitors record proportionately greater time on screening than practice nurses – 19% compared to 8% – which may account for this). Further analyses reveal that the two groups of nurses carry out the activity of health education in different locations: practice nurses on surgery premises and health visitors in clients' homes (and similarly for the location of the activity of treatment carried out by practice nurses and district nurses). This finding may be of significance in future health-care delivery patterns.

Currently there is much discussion about future UK general practice being focused along the lines of health maintenance organizations in the USA with patients being seen for all but a fraction of their care on surgery premises, virtually eliminating domiciliary visits and conducting all procedures on surgery premises. If this scenario were to unfold in the UK, then the location of some of the activities recorded by these groups of community nurses becomes important and the issue of 'overlap of activities', although not relevant in the current climate, may indeed become a focus of attention for future rationalization.

Delegation – enhancing roles or shedding unpleasant tasks?

The notion of delegation in general practice is not new. For example, Robinson (1990) drew attention to this as a way for GPs to cope with their ever-increasing workloads, adding that delegation is most likely to be aimed at nurses because much of the workload increase is within their scope. The study described here provides the evidence for this forecast – evidence generated by GPs themselves – that a not inconsiderable proportion of their work could be referred on to other members of the PHCT.

Reference was made earlier to the use of the term 'delegation' as opposed to the term 'referral'. The former term suggests that work is being transferred from one member of the PHCT to another, usually from a doctor to a nurse, and hence this carries with it the notion of delegating down. A more equitable term may be 'allocation of work' which suggests that all members of the PHCT operate on an equal footing. The change of vocabulary here may not be greeted with approval by the medical profession at the present time but its introduction represents a logical step forward.

The findings from our study indicating that 39% of consultations had a delegatable element and that 17% of all consultations could be passed on in their entirety to someone else is only the beginning of the story. Mechanisms need to be identified and implemented; examples do exist, but at present they are being implemented in an *ad hoc* fashion. Triage in general practice would facilitate these opportunities but this still begs the question of who would be the most appropriate professional to carry out this function. Such speculation raises the question of liability. Similarly, the formulation of protocols carries with it the same drawbacks. In addition, are protocols themselves truly a team effort or are they driven by doctors?

This study also identifies the activities most amenable to delegation to both practice nurses and nurse practitioners. That the single most oft-quoted activity is that of advice and reassurance is interesting and begs further investigation. Could it be that (mainly male) doctors perceive (mainly female) nurses as the more caring gender and therefore better able to undertake this activity? Or is it that doctors perceive nurses as having more time to spend with patients than themselves in busy surgeries?

CONCLUSION

The workload and labour force crisis in general practice described earlier is here to stay and the evidence provided by our study demonstrates that there are ways of alleviating some of the problems. In all the practices participating in this study, delegation and teamwork represent acceptable modes of delivering primary care. By effective teamworking, allocation of workload suggests equitable, integrated working by interprofessional teams. Phrases such as 'Some GP groups now use well-trained nurses to diagnose and treat patients' (Maynard 1997) may yet become redundant.

Whilst one would not deny that there are reservations about the process of delegation, these should not necessarily be seen negatively. Disputes about roles and boundaries and practice nurses being handmaidens to their GP colleagues of course should be aired but should not influence the future. Skill mix should be seen in a more positive light – one concerned with getting the balance 'right' in primary-care delivery – about care being given to patients by people who are best qualified and most appropriate to deliver it, about people working together in teams, and about a willingness to look to the future.

At the heart of the two White Papers, Choice and Opportunity (Department of Health 1996a) and Delivering the Future (Department of Health 1996b), lies the concept of flexibility. In order to bring the two concepts of skill mix and flexibility into the debate, consideration of the notion of balance, central to this chapter, is essential. These two White Papers present community nursing with lots of opportunities for increasing the influence of nursing on the delivery of primary care in the future. These are exciting and exhilarating times and a challenge to all community nurses. The challenge is one of real partnerships with GP colleagues and of accepting enhanced roles (with due caution) in order that nurses working in primary care can play an active part in changing the culture of the delivery of primary care.

QUESTIONS FOR DISCUSSION

◆ What tasks should only be provided by GPs?

◆ What tasks could be delegated to others, under supervision?

◆ What tasks could be delegated to others, without supervision?

ANNOTATED BIBLIOGRAPHY

Atkin K, Lunt N, Parker G, Hirst M 1993 Nurses count. A national census of practice nurses. Social Policy Research Unit, University of York

This book presents data from a national census of practice nurses (see Chapter 7, this volume). Of particular relevance to this chapter is its account of the work undertaken by practice nurses as part of their daily routine.

Jenkins-Clarke S, Carr-Hill R 1996 Measuring skill mix in primary care: dilemmas of delegation and diversification. Discussion Paper 144. Centre for Health Economics, University of York

This discussion paper outlines the issues informing the measurement of skill mix in primary care and the difficulties that emerge.

Acknowledgements

The York study described in this chapter was funded by the Department of Health; the views expressed here are those of the author alone. The research team comprised Sue Jenkins-Clarke, Roy Carr-Hill, Paul Dixon (at the Centre for Health Economics, University of York) and Mike Pringle (Professor of General Practice, University of Nottingham). Barbara Duncan was a research fellow from January 1995 to March 1996. In total there were five research nurses who undertook data collection at the sites on a rota basis: Elizabeth Allen, Jill Carley, Christine Dowell, Ann Richards and Bridget Smith. The project could not have been undertaken without the help and cooperation of all the community nurses, practice managers, secretarial and clerical staff and GPs at the sites we visited. To them I am most grateful; without exception they welcomed us into their premises, allowed us to document details of their working lives for 2 weeks and suffered the consequent disruption with equanimity.

REFERENCES

Atkin K, Lunt N 1993 A census of direction. Nursing Times 89 (42): 38–40
Atkin K, Lunt M 1995 Nurses in practice: the role of the practice nurse in primary health care. Social Policy Research Unit, University of York
Bagust A, Slack R, Oakley J 1992 Ward nursing quality and grade mix. Report of paired ward experiment undertaken in the North West Region. York Health Economics Consortium, University of York
Bowling A 1981 Delegation to nurses in general practice. Journal of the Royal College of General Practitioners 31: 485–490
Carr E, Kirk B, Jeffcoate W 1991 Perceived needs of general practitioners and practice nurses for the care of diabetic patients. Diabetic medicine 8: 556–559
Carr-Hill R A, Dixon P, Gibbs I et al 1992 Skill mix and the effectiveness of nursing care. Centre For Health Economics, University of York
Charlton I, Charlton G, Broomfield J, Mullee M 1991 Audit on the effect of a nurse run asthma clinic on workload and patient morbidity in a general practice. British journal of general practice 41: 227–231
Denton F T, Gafni A, Spencer B G, Stoddart G L 1983 Potential savings from the adoption of nurse practitioners in the Canadian health care system. Socio-econ plan sci 17 (4): 199–209
Department of Health 1992 The health of the nation. HMSO, London
Department of Health and NHS Management Executive 1994 NHS workforce in England 1981–1991. BAOSS (Health Publications Unit), No. 2 site, Manchester
Department of Health 1995 Planning the medical workforce. Medical workforce standing advisory committee: second report. Department of Health, London
Department of Health 1996a Choice and opportunity. Primary care: the future. The Stationery Office, London

Department of Health 1996b Primary care: delivering the future. The Stationery Office, London

Georgian Research Society 1991 The attitudes of general practitioners towards practice nurses: A pilot study. British journal of general practice 41: 19–22

Handysides S 1994 Morale in general practice: is change the problem or the solution? British medical journal 308: 32–34

Jenkins-Clarke S, Carr-Hill R A 1996 Measuring skill mix in primary care: dilemmas of delegation and diversification. Discussion paper No. 144. University of York, Centre for Health Economics, York

Jenkins-Clarke S, Carr-Hill R A, Dixon P, Pringle M 1997 Skills mix in primary care. Final report. Centre for Health Economics, York

Jewell D, Hope J 1988 Evaluation of a nurse run hypertension clinic in general practice. Practitioner 232: 484–487

Leigh M 1996 The doc brief, nineties-style. The Guardian, March 13: 10

Lloyd M, Webb S, Singh S 1994 Community care reforms: early implications for general practice. British journal of general practice 44 (385): 338–339

Marsh G, Dawes M 1995 Establishing a minor illness nurse in a busy general practice. British medical journal 310: 778–780

Maynard A 1997 Wringing out the wets. Health service journal 107 (5557): 25

McBride M, Metcalfe D 1995 General practitioners' low morale: reasons and solutions. British journal of general practice 145: 227–229

McKenna H P 1995 Nursing skill mix substitutions and quality of care: an exploration of assumptions from the research literature. Journal of advanced nursing 21 (3): 452–459

Nessling R 1990 Manpower monograph (No. 2). Skill mix: a practical approach for health professionals. Department of Health/MPAG, London

NHS Management Executive, Value For Money Unit 1992 The nursing skill mix in the district nursing service. HMSO, London

Robinson G 1990 The future for practice nurses. British journal of general practice 40: 132–133

Robinson G, Beaton S, White P 1993 Attitudes towards practice nurses: survey of a sample of general practitioners in England and Wales. British journal of general practice 43: 25–29

Salisbury C, Tettersall M 1988 Comparison of the work of the nurse practitioner with that of the general practitioner. Journal of the Royal College of General Practitioners 38: 314–316

Seccombe I, Patch A, Stock J 1994 Workloads, pay and morale of qualified nurses in 1994. Report 272. Institute of Manpower Studies, London

Spitzer W O, Sackett D L, Sibley J C et al 1974 The Burlington randomised trial of the nurse practitioner. New England Journal of Medicine 290: 251–256

Stilwell B, Greenfield S, Drury M, Hull F 1987 A nurse practitioner in general practice: working style and pattern of consultations. Journal of the Royal College of General Practitioners 37: 154–157

Wade B 1993 The job satisfaction of health visitors, district nurses and practice nurses working in areas served by four trusts: Year 1. Journal of Advanced Nursing 18: 992–1004

4

Prescribing and community nursing – an evaluation of practice

Karen Luker   Lynn Austin

KEY ISSUES

- The benefits of nurse prescribing have been advocated for more than two decades.
- Legislation permitting nurses in England to prescribe came into place in October 1994.
- An evaluation of nurse prescribing in the first eight demonstration sites found positive benefits for patients, carers and health-care professionals.
- National expansion of nurse prescribing is a policy reality.

INTRODUCTION

The arguments in favour of nurse prescribing have been debated for many years. This chapter charts the history of nurse prescribing from the late 1970s, when the debate focused on prescribing by nurses working in family planning services, to the present date where it seems likely that nurse prescribing will be implemented on a national basis. Key reports during this time are detailed along with the main findings from a Department of Health-funded evaluation of this new initiative. The chapter ends by considering the implications of nurse prescribing for practice and management.

The debate concerning prescribing rights for nurses spans more than two decades. Much of the early literature focused on the prescribing of contraceptives by nurses providing family planning services (DHSS 1976, RCN 1980). Following the publication of the Cumberlege Report (DHSS 1986) the debate widened. The remit of the working party, chaired by Baroness Cumberlege, was to study the nursing services provided by health authorities to people living at home and how these services could be used more effectively. A number of recommendations were made, including the introduction of the nurse practitioner role into the community. Limited prescribing rights were also seen to be essential if nurses were to work effectively and it was proposed that:

> *The DHSS should agree a limited list of items and simple agents which may be prescribed by nurses as part of a nursing care programme, and issue guidelines to enable nurses to control drug dosage in well defined circumstances.* (DHSS 1986)

In response to this recommendation, the Department of Health established a working party (Department of Health 1989a) to determine the extent to which nurse prescribing could benefit patients cared for in their own home. The working party's recommendations, disseminated in the Crown Report, suggested that nurses with a district nurse (DN) or health visitor (HV) qualification, following the necessary additional training, should be:

> *... empowered to prescribe items for patients with those conditions for which the nurse takes independent clinical responsibility.* (Department of Health 1989a)

Three forms of prescribing were proposed to enable nurses to manage a patient's condition more effectively and these are outlined in Box 4.1. Initial prescribing by nurses was advocated solely for nurses with a DN or HV qualification. However, the supply of medicines in accordance with group or patient-specific protocols was considered appropriate for other nurses who had undertaken further specialist education, training and assessment: for example, continence advisers, specialist nurses for terminally ill patients and diabetic liaison nurses. The Crown Report (Department of Health 1989a), whilst making specific recommendations, considered that the issue of nurse prescribing required further review, in particular, the extension of prescribing rights to other groups of specialist nurses and the addition of further items to the Nurses' Formulary. The need for an evaluation of both the cost and

---

Box 4.1 Forms of nurse prescribing

◆ Initial prescribing by nurses from a Nurses' Formulary.

◆ Supplying within a group protocol agreed for a clinical service (e.g. vaccinations, stoma items by stoma care nurses).

◆ Adjusting the timing and dosage of medicines prescribed by medical practitioners within a patient-specific protocol (e.g. specialist nurses).

benefits of the nurses' new role was also highlighted; this was to include an assessment of the views of patients, carers, nurses and other members of the primary health-care team (PHCT) in addition to economic appraisal.

Whilst awaiting the legislative changes required to enact the recommendations contained within the Crown Report, the Department of Health commissioned Touche Ross to undertake a study examining the likely impact of nurse prescribing (Department of Health 1991). It sought to identify the costs and benefits of nurse prescribing by gathering data (via interview and questionnaires) from a number of respondents including community nurses, general practitioners (GPs) and pharmacists. The study reported widespread support for the principle of nurse prescribing and found that many nurses in the community generated scripts signed by GPs without significant challenge to their recommendation, on the grounds of either cost or appropriateness. The main benefits anticipated were small weekly time savings for patients, nurses and GPs, although it was considered unlikely that this would translate into reduced expenditure due to the fragmented nature of the time saved. Further unquantified benefits anticipated included faster access to items by patients and increased job satisfaction for nurses.

The primary legislation to enable nurses to prescribe (the Medicinal Products Prescription by Nurses Act 1992) was passed on 16 March 1992. The legislative vehicle was a private member's bill, which the government approved. The necessary commencement order and secondary legislation came into force in October 1994. An amendment to the Pharmaceutical Services and Charges for Drugs and Appliances Regulations also came into force in October 1994 to allow pharmacists to dispense nurse-prescribed medicines.

Organizational changes

Following the announcement by Baroness Cumberlege that an evaluation to determine the feasibility of nurse prescribing was to take place, a letter was sent to each of the eight newly formed regional health authorities (NHS Executive 1994). This asked them to contact fundholders in their region and invite applications from practices wishing to participate in the evaluation. Practices were required to fulfil a number of criteria in order to be considered for inclusion. Regions were asked to produce a shortlist of three interested sites and forward the details to the NHS Executive. Sites were ultimately selected by the Department of Health so that the overall sample included a mix of features, including location (rural or urban), practice size and wave of fundholding.

In order to be entered onto the professional list of nurse prescribers, nurses had to complete an English National Board (ENB)-approved training course (ENB 1992). Nurses eligible to prescribe at each of the demonstration sites, including practice nurses (PNs) with a DN or HV qualification, undertook training in nurse prescribing in accordance with the guidelines laid down by the ENB. This consisted of an open learning pack and a 2-day taught component. The open learning pack was estimated to take 15 h to complete and covered a number of areas including prescribing safely and effectively, accountability and ethical issues. The main aim of the precourse material was to bring all nurses up to the same educational level for the start of the prescribing course which built on the knowledge gained from the open learning pack. Course topics included pharmacology, generic prescribing and the legal and ethical issues of prescribing. At the end of the second day nurses completed an assessment which took the form of a written examination. Of the 60 participating nurses, 58 successfully completed the nurse prescribing training course.

Organizational changes required to implement the enabling legislation included the production of prescription pads for prescribing nurses, which were colour coded green for DNs and HVs and lilac for PNs. The colours facilitated identification of scripts by the Prescription Pricing Authority (PPA), the organization responsible for handling NHS prescriptions. The United Kingdom Central Council (UKCC) also permitted pharmacists access to the 'voicebank' in order that verification of a nurse's prescribing status could be obtained.

A Nurse Prescribers' Formulary (NPF) (BMA et al 1994) was produced which included items required by nurses as part of their day-to-day care of patients, for example, wound and skin-care products, mild analgesics, laxatives and treatment for oral candidiasis. The majority of prescribable items were available over the counter (OTC) although six categories of prescription-only medicines (POMs) were added to the NPF 3 months after the implementation of nurse prescribing

EVALUATING PRESCRIBING PRACTICE

Impact on service delivery

The potential changes in service delivery, once nurse prescribing was implemented, were detailed in the Crown Report (Department of Health 1989a), the Touche Ross study (Department of Health 1991) and the nursing press (Poulton 1994, Shuttleworth 1994). The main changes anticipated were savings in time for patients, carers, nurses and other health-care professionals. These changes were confirmed by nurses participating in the Department of Health evaluation (Luker et al 1996a,b,c). Whilst time savings were undoubtedly a consideration, nurses were also likely to report the convenience of being able to instigate treatment immediately.

Nurses considered themselves to be in a position to prescribe NPF items more cost effectively than GPs. This was related to a number of factors:

◆ the emphasis placed on generic prescribing;

- nurses' increased awareness of the cost of similar products, now they were referring to a formulary;
- familiarity with the pack sizes for items such as wound-care products, permitting nurses to tailor the prescription to the patient's needs;
- the nurses' close contact with patients which ensured that patients did not stockpile items at home.

Nurses' reports that they were able to prescribe more cost effectively than GPs were interesting given the concern expressed that cost containment would be the overriding factor when it came to assessing the success of nurse prescribing (Shuttleworth 1994). The extent to which this heightened awareness of costs was a result of nurses feeling under close scrutiny is not known.

The information provided to patients by nurses when issuing a prescription for NPF items was considered, by two-thirds of the nurses in the evaluation, to be better than that provided by GPs. This perception was also held by half of the GPs interviewed and to a lesser extent by patients – 13% thought the information provided was better but none thought it was worse. In general, nurses were considered to give more detailed information thereby enabling the patient to use the prescribed item more effectively.

Improvements in service delivery were noted by many patients. Obtaining a prescription directly from the nurse had resulted in DN patients, in particular, receiving items more promptly and being less dependent on others to obtain items on their behalf. Some patients required items on a repeat prescription basis and, in the past, this necessitated requesting the items, obtaining the prescription and having the item dispensed at the chemist, a procedure which could take over 48 h. Some of these stages had now been omitted, resulting in easier access to prescribed items.

The service had improved for HV clients as they no longer had to consult another professional to obtain prescriptions for problems which could be managed by the HV. This was particularly beneficial given that gaining access to the HV was generally more straightforward than making an appointment to see the GP and attending the surgery. This resulted in some clients reporting health-related problems – such as skin rash – to the HV which they would not necessarily have presented to the GP.

Whilst nurse prescribing had resulted in a more responsive service for patients, a small number (13%) were unaware that the nurse was able to prescribe. This, however, simply emphasizes the efforts nurses previously made to provide a service for patients. Prior to nurse prescribing nurses commonly obtained prescribed items on the patient's behalf or arranged for the chemist to deliver items, the patient often not seeing the actual prescription. The only change that had taken place for the patients was that the nurse now signed the prescription instead of the GP.

Impact on professional roles

The introduction of nurse prescribing has resulted in nurses encroaching on areas traditionally considered to be the province of doctors. Diagnosis and medical treatment have always been seen as central to medical authority (Sweet & Norman 1995). Nurses assuming responsibility for some areas of the prescribing domain may be perceived by some as a threat to the professionalism and status of the GP. Whilst the impact of nurse prescribing on professional relationships is difficult to ascertain at present, especially given the fact that those interviewed in this evaluation volunteered to be demonstration sites, there are indications that not all GPs view this development in a positive light (GP 1995).

The experience of nurse prescribing in other countries suggests that some doctors are opposed to it, leading them to emphasize what could happen if things go wrong. District nurses and HVs in Sweden have been prescribing dressings and appliances for around 20 years. The Swedish formulary was extended in October 1994 allowing a range of oral medications to be prescribed. Swedish nurses, after completing an 8-week training course, can now prescribe 230 brands of products for 60 specific indications (David & Brown 1995). However, some doctors considered that 8 weeks was insufficient for nurses to learn how to diagnose correctly and there were fears that more serious conditions would be missed (Enkat om distriktsskoterskors forshrinningsratt 1994). This resulted in the doctors highlighting rare cases where diagnosis could be problematic; for example, although discomfort around the anus is usually harmless, cancer of the rectum may be a possibility.

The Crown Report (Department of Health 1989a) noted that nurse prescribing would help clarify professional responsibilities and strengthen relationships between nurses and their colleagues. Both this report and the Touche Ross study (Department of Health 1991) acknowledged that nurses were already making treatment decisions for patients which the GP simply endorsed. Overall, nurses interviewed for the Department of Health evaluation (Luker et al 1996a) reported that their ability to work independently of the GP resulted in higher levels of job satisfaction, primarily as nurses were now seen to be responsible for decisions made. GPs also expressed confidence in nurses' ability to prescribe NPF items. Consequently, none of the nurses had their prescribing decisions challenged by a GP.

Not only are treatment decisions made by nurses largely unchallenged by GPs, it has been argued that nurses actually influence GPs' prescribing behaviour, most notably for wound-care products, an area in which some GPs are considered less knowledgeable than nurses (Nursing Standard 1990). This perception was also held by nurses and GPs in the Department of Health evaluation (Luker et al 1996a). Work undertaken by the Royal College of Nursing (RCN 1995) suggests that, for PNs, this influence extends to products not included in the NPF, for example, asthma treatments and contraceptives. This has led some to call for extensions to the NPF so that it better reflects nurses' areas of activity.

The role of nurses working in the community has changed considerably since the Crown Report's recommendations (Department of Health 1989a), most notably as a result of the reform of the health service after the implementation of the NHS and Community Care Act 1990 and its increasing emphasis on the care of patients in the community. It is perhaps not surprising that the implementation of only one aspect of prescribing – initial prescribing – proposed in the Report is seen as inadequate by some groups.

It is the role of the PN which has changed most since the Crown Report with the number of PNs working in primary care showing a steady increase for a number of years (Atkin et al 1993). It is not just the number of PNs that has changed, but the nature of their work. Recent studies have shown that PNs now take responsibility for a variety of different areas outside the traditional treatment room (Bentley 1991, Atkin et al 1993; also Chapter 7, this volume). The GP contract of 1990 (Department of Health 1989b) was a catalyst for many of these changes due to the increasing emphasis placed on the need for health checks. In many cases work has been delegated to PNs by GPs, in some instances supported by the use of guidelines or protocols. The recommendations with regard to protocols, contained within the Crown Report, were therefore superseded to some extent by practice developments which had taken place prior to the implementation of legislative changes. It is noteworthy that this is now an area subject to some controversy as the legality of protocols in relation to the supply of medicines has come under close scrutiny (Naish 1996).

Impact on preparation

At present only PNs with a DN or HV qualification are eligible to become nurse prescribers. This is due, in part, to the perceived need for nurses to have a further recordable qualification to act as a benchmark with regard to their level of knowledge (Bentley 1991). However, only 14% of PNs have such a qualification (Atkin et al 1993). The views of respondents in the nurse-prescribing evaluation varied with respect to which categories of nurse should be permitted to prescribe, although it was generally agreed that nurse prescribing should be implemented in other sites. Nurses seemed to fall into two camps with regard to extending nurse prescribing to PNs or other specialist nurses. For some, the possession of a DN or HV qualification was seen as important, as was the need for some experience in this area of work. Others viewed the exclusion of PNs as inappropriate as these nurses were considered to have the necessary knowledge to prescribe. The level of training and expertise held by some specialist nurses, for example those working with patients with asthma or diabetes, was also seen by some as a justification for extending prescribing rights. Although some GPs commented that a dual qualification should be necessary to become a prescriber, they did not consider that this should only be for DNs or HVs. In particular, many GPs were concerned about the exclusion of PNs not holding a DN or HV qualification.

The training of PNs is an important point and relevant to nurse prescribing. Atkin et al (1993) found the training of PNs to be variable and less than half of their sample, represented in a national census, had attended a course validated by one of the national boards. However, it is noteworthy that a strategy is in place, endorsed by the United Kingdom Central Council (UKCC 1996) for practice nurses to have their previous studies recognized without the requirement to complete a further programme of education, provided that they can demonstrate that they have met the outcomes of a recordable programme of at least 16 weeks (full-time equivalent). The ENB A51 practice nursing programme meets the UKCC requirements in this respect. Therefore PNs who so wish may complete and present a comprehensive portfolio of previous learning for assessment against the outcomes of the ENB A51 programme. Practice nurses choosing this route, on successful assessment, would be recommended by the approved educational institution to the ENB for the A51 award so they can record this on the UKCC register and then use the title of specialist practitioner. This has implications for the future preparation of nurses for prescribing. If PNs are seen to have a further registerable qualification this negates some of the arguments against prescribing rights for this group of nurses. The training needs of PNs also receive attention in the Department of Health White Paper Primary Care: Delivering the Future (Department of Health 1996a). This suggests that health authorities should work closely with GPs and primary-care teams to identify practice nurses' requirements for induction programmes, education and training. The need for professional support and mentorship of PNs is stressed, therefore good practice guidelines are to be produced to assist health authorities and GPs produce development programmes for PNs (see also Chapter 7).

In addition to the debate around who should be trained, the method whereby nurses receive training also requires consideration. Prescribing nurses in the Department of Health evaluation (Luker et al 1996a) offered many useful comments as to how the nurse-prescribing training could be modified to best meet their needs. These included the length of the course, the content of the training programme and the format of assessment. Further consideration as to when this training should take place and how it could be funded is necessary. Some view the incorporation of nurse prescribing into the general training of nurses undertaking the DN or HV certificate as appropriate. Others view the establishment of specific training courses as the preferred option. Whichever method is selected, there will be a need for continual update although opinions may differ as to where responsibilities lie. A balance needs to be struck between the responsibility of the nurse and the employer regarding clinical update. This is not restricted to nurse prescribing but is part of the necessary culture change if evidence-based practice is to become a reality. Postregistration education and practice (PREP) requires nurses to undertake 5 study days in 3 years and this could be one way of updating prescribing nurses.

The issue of funding for training also requires resolution if nurse prescribing is to be adopted on a national basis. Funding was a concern of community nurse managers and GPs at the evaluation sites. Some considered that it should be a joint responsibility between the community trust/unit and the GP practice whereas others viewed national funding as the preferred option.

IMPLICATIONS FOR PRACTICE AND MANAGEMENT

Following a long campaign by nurses, nurse prescribing is now a reality even though it is in a more limited guise than that envisaged by the Crown Report (Department of Health 1989a). Only one aspect of nurse prescribing – initial prescribing from a formulary – has been fully evaluated. This can be attributed, in part, to the fact that many ideas contained within the Crown Report, most notably prescribing in accordance with protocols, were superseded by changes taking place within nursing and primary-care services, in particular the developing role of PNs and nurse practitioners who, in many cases, have taken on aspects of work traditionally undertaken by GPs. Where this has required the provision of prescription-only medicines, the development of guidelines has taken place. The legality of guidelines and protocols has now come under close scrutiny.

The changing role of nurses has led some to argue that prescribing rights should be extended to those who do not possess a DN or HV qualification. The recent attempts to ensure that PNs are able to obtain a registerable qualification may lend weight to this argument. The issue of who is to be trained and, equally, who will fund the training and where it will take place is yet to be determined. The idea of extending the NPF has also been advanced as this would facilitate the progression of nurse prescribing. It is suggested that the current NPF no longer reflects the areas of work in which nurses take primary responsibility.

The evaluation study of nurse prescribing (Luker et al 1996a) demonstrated that initial prescribing by nurses was a success and fulfilled many of the pre-prescribing expectations. Further evaluative work is now underway in one community unit (Department of Health 1996b) and the government (Department of Health 1996a) has recently announced that the current nurse-prescribing scheme was to be extended to a further seven NHS trusts, one in each of the remaining regions in England, with a view to full implementation in April 1998. However, the expansion of nurse prescribing has not occurred as expected in April 1998, although the Health Secretary has expressed a commitment to full roll out.

In the interim a further review of the prescribing, supply and administration of medicines is underway and there are indications that prescribing may be extended to other specialist nurses (DoH 1997). An interim report has been published (DoH 1998) regarding prescribing by group protocol. This suggests that while prescribing in accordance with group protocols may be necessary in limited circumstances, criteria should be in place to ensure that this is undertaken safely. These developments should go some way towards alleviating the concerns expressed regarding the limited nature of nurse prescribing and permitting nurses to demonstrate the true potential of this new role.

CONCLUSION

Nurse prescribing was viewed as an undoubted success by those participating in the evaluation. It will be interesting to note whether or not the benefits noted at the eight demonstration sites are experienced by other sites or whether new factors emerge as a result of this extension.

QUESTIONS FOR DISCUSSION

◆ To what extent, if any, should the Nurse Prescribers' Formulary be extended?

◆ Should there be a separate formulary for nurses or should nurses have access to the full range of items in the British National Formulary (BNF) and prescribe items which they consider themselves competent to prescribe and which relate to the nursing aspects of patient care?

◆ What form should the training of nurses in relation to prescribing take? Should it be part of the core training of nurses working in the community or should it be a specific course?

◆ Who should fund the training for nurse prescribing? Is this a practice, trust or national responsibility?

◆ Should specialist nurses be permitted to prescribe?

◆ Do you think nurse prescribing requires nurses to make a diagnosis and if so, do you think this is appropriate?

ANNOTATED BIBLIOGRAPHY

Luker K, Austin L, Willock J, Ferguson B, Smith K 1997 Nurses' and GPs' views of the nurse prescribers' formulary. Nursing Standard 11 (22): 33–38

This paper presents findings from the evaluation of nurse prescribing and focuses on the types of items nurses and GPs would like to see incorporated into the NPF and the limitations of the formulary in its present form.

Luker K, Austin L, Hogg C, Ferguson B, Smith K 1997 Nurse prescribing: the views of nurses and other health care professionals. British Journal of Community Health Nursing 2 (2): 69–74

This paper presents findings from the evaluation of nurse prescribing and focuses on the views of health-care professionals at the eight demonstration sites including the type of items prescribed and advantages and disadvantages noted in relation to the nurses' new role.

Luker K, Hogg C, Austin L, Ferguson B, Smith K 1997 Over the counter items bought by a sample of community nurse patients. British Journal of Community Health Nursing 2 (2): 75–82

This paper presents findings from the evaluation of nurse prescribing and focuses on the behaviour of patients in relation to the purchase of OTC items and whether this had been affected by the nurse's ability to prescribe items from a formulary (the majority of which are available to buy OTC). The findings are compared to those of similar studies examining self-medication.

REFERENCES

Atkin K, Lunt N, Parker G, Hirst M 1993 Nurses count: a national census of practice nurses. SPRU, University of York

Bentley H 1991 Back to the future. Nursing Times 87 (24): 29–31

British Medical Association, Royal Pharmaceutical Society of Great Britain, Health Visitors Association and Royal College of Nursing 1994 Nurse prescribers' formulary 1994 (pilot edition). British Medical Association, Royal Pharmaceutical Society of Great Britain in association with the Health Visitors Association and Royal College of Nursing, London

David A, Brown E 1995 How Swedish nurses are tackling nurse prescribing. Nursing times 91 (50): 23–44

Department of Health 1989a Report of the advisory group on nurse prescribing (Crown report). HMSO, London

Department of Health 1989b General practice in the National Health Service – the 1990 contract. HMSO, London

Department of Health 1991 Nurse prescribing final report: a cost benefit study (Touche Ross report). HMSO, London

Department of Health 1996a Primary care: delivering the future. HMSO, London

Department of Health 1996b Lady Cumberlege announces extension to nurse prescribing (press release 18 January). HMSO, London

Department of Health 1997 Review of prescribing, supply and administration of medicines. NHS Executive, Leeds

Department of Health 1998 Review of prescribing, supply and administrations of medicines: report on the supply and administration of medicines under group protocol. NHS Executive, Leeds

Department of Health and Social Security 1976 Report of the joint working group on oral contraceptives. HMSO, London

Department of Health and Social Security 1986 Neighbourhood nursing: a focus for care (Cumberlege report). HMSO, London

English National Board 1992 Nurse prescribing: guidelines for the preparation of district nurses and health visitors (Circular 1992/30/MB). English National Board, London

Enkat Om Distriktsskoterskors Forshrinningsratt 1994 Vanskligt att uppfylla kravey pa rayt diagnos. Lakartidningen 91 (28–29): 2694–2698

General Practitioner 1995 Are nurses more valued than GPs? GP 6 October: 48

Luker K A, Ferguson B, Austin L et al 1996a Evaluation of nurse prescribing: final report. Department of Health, Leeds

Luker K A, Austin L, Hogg C, Ferguson B, Smith K 1996b Nurse prescribing: the views of nurses and other health care professionals. British Journal of Community Health Nursing 2 (2): 69–74

Luker K A, Austin L, Hogg C, Ferguson B, Smith K 1996c Patients' views of nurse prescribing: findings from the evaluation. Nursing Times Vol 93 no 17

Naish J 1996 Prescribed confusion. Nursing Times 92 (49): 56

NHS Executive 1994 Nurse prescribing EL(94)31. NHS Executive, London

Nursing Standard 1990 Educated for change. Nursing standard 4 (44)(suppl): 13

Poulton B C 1994 Nurse prescribing. Broadening the scope of professional practice. International nursing review 41 (3): 81–84

Royal College of Nursing 1980 Nurse prescribers of oral contraceptives for the well woman. Royal College of Nursing, London

Royal College of Nursing 1995 Whose prescription? Royal College of Nursing, London

Shuttleworth A 1994 Prescribing trial must have a fighting chance. Professional Nurse (editorial) 9 (4): 220

Sweet S, Norman I 1995 The nurse–doctor relationship: a selective literature review: Journal of advanced nursing 22: 165–174

United Kingdom Central Council 1996 The council's standards for education and practice following registration (PREP): transitional arrangements – specialist practitioner title/specialist qualification. United Kingdom Central Council, London

Section 2

Evaluating changes to practice arenas

5. School nursing – an evaluation of policy and practice   *79*

6. Evaluation and community psychiatric nursing   *107*

7. The emergence and development of practice nursing – implications for future policy and practice   *129*

8. Evaluating learning disability – embracing change   *153*

5

School nursing – an evaluation of policy and practice

Wendy Bines   Jane Lightfoot

KEY ISSUES

- School nursing is an 'invisible' service, with much of its contribution to child health hidden.

- Although school nurses are uniquely placed to gather a wide range of information about the health of the school-age population, the potential for using this information to target services and shape commissioning is underdeveloped.

- School nurses could play a greater part in facilitating children's voices to be heard by those responsible for commissioning and planning services.

INTRODUCTION

This chapter evaluates key policy developments in the health service in relation to current and potential roles of school nurses. This policy evaluation is grounded in empirical research findings, drawn from a study commissioned by the Department of Health to examine the role of nursing for school-age children (Lightfoot & Bines 1997). School nursing is an important case study, since it illuminates the impact of policy change on a branch of community health nursing which, for a variety of reasons, has remained relatively hidden from wider view and scrutiny.

The hidden nature of school nursing has four main dimensions:

- School nursing is part of the school health service, described by Harrison & Gretton (1986) as the 'invisible' service. School health services have low priority in national policy terms, subjected only to limited statutory requirements and national guidance. In turn, the low priority accorded to school health services influences the status of those professionals who deliver the service.

◆ School nursing is a low-profile workforce. School nurses are few in number: although central government no longer collates data on the number of school nurses nationally, evidence suggests there were around 2350 nurses in post in England in 1994 (House of Commons Health Committee 1997, p. xi–xii).

◆ Due to limited educational requirements and opportunities, school nursing has achieved lower professional status than other groups of community health nurses.

◆ The low profile of school nurses is compounded by the fact that most of their work takes place outside typical NHS settings, risking both isolation from and marginalization by NHS colleagues.

These factors underpin the implications of wider policy changes (see Chapter 1) for school nursing, which the chapter tackles in a number of sections. Initially, three key policy themes are identified and their relevance to school nursing established. We then use our empirical research evidence to investigate both the current and potential role of the school nurse against the context of these policy developments. Separate sections follow, focusing on the implications of policy developments for the education and preparation of nurses working with school-age children and for evaluating services. In our conclusion, we reflect on the position of school nursing as a result of these policy developments and in the light of our evidence. The remainder of this introductory section provides background information on our research, on the school health service and on school nursing.

The research project

This chapter presents empirical data collected by the authors in a study for the Department of Health on the role of nursing in meeting the health needs of school-age children outside hospital (Lightfoot & Bines 1997). Given the lack of previous research in this field, the project was exploratory in character and sought to generate information about the role of nursing in meeting health needs common to all children, such as health promotion and the prevention of illness. The study inevitably, but not exclusively, turned to the work of school nurses, who have a dedicated role for this client group. Specifically, the project had eight objectives:

◆ To identify the normative health status of school-age children.
◆ To identify national priorities for community and primary health services for school-age children.

◆ To investigate the contribution of nursing in meeting health needs, both in terms of the broad role of nurses and specific activities carried out by them.

◆ To explore the interface between nursing and other professions in meeting children's health needs, including with whom nurses liaise, collaborate and communicate and in what circumstances.

◆ To examine nurses' work in partnership with children and their parents.

◆ To examine how responsibilities for meeting community and primary health needs of children not in school are managed.

◆ To examine factors which appear to influence the role of nurses, including the constraints and opportunities facing nurses in meeting children's health needs.

◆ To suggest possible explanations for any variations in nursing practice.

Empirical research was carried out in four health authority sites. The study used semistructured interviews with 24 school nurses, 18 other community health nurses and 27 heads and teachers and 36 interviews with health commissioners, managers and local authority staff. Seven discussion groups were held with parents and eight groups with young people. Qualitative methods were considered appropriate for this exploratory study to gather rich accounts from respondents and so gain valuable insights into current nursing practice.

The school health service

The school health service has its roots in the development of state education and the public health movement (Harris 1995). Following the 1870 Education Act, the introduction of compulsory elementary education exposed 'the extent of malnutrition, ill health and physical defects among the school aged population' (Vine 1991). After the turn of the century child health became a national concern, not least because of the high rate of potential recruits for the Boer War rejected due to ill health (While & Barriball 1993, British Pediatric Association 1995). The Education Act 1907 required 'periodic medical inspections' of children of elementary school age and marked the beginnings of a universal school health service.

Until 1974, when responsibility for the school health service passed to health authorities, the service was in the hands of local education authorities (LEAs). The 1944 Education Act gave LEAs the duty to carry out medical and dental inspections of school children, provide free treatment and to ascertain children needing 'special' education. Following the introduction of the NHS in 1948, treatment services gradually passed to GPs and to hospital services, with the school health service retaining preventive and advisory roles. The Education Acts of 1981 and 1993 have continued to specify requirements and offer guidance concerning the role of the school health service for children with special educational needs. However, the only statutory requirements governing the universal school health service remain those in the NHS Act 1977 for medical and dental inspections of school children attending maintained (now including grant maintained) schools 'at appropriate intervals' (para 5 (1) (a)). There is, however, no definitive guidance as to the role, content, staffing (or setting!) of the service.

In its recent guidance on good practice in child health services in the community, the Department of Health urges the school health service to be considered as part of 'a comprehensive service to meet the health needs of school-age children', including members of primary health-care teams (PHCTs), teachers and parents. The broad aims of such a service are twofold: 'to promote the physical and mental health of school-age children' and 'to enable children to achieve their educational potential' (Department of Health 1996, para 8.1). The more specific objectives set by the Department of Health for the school health service indicate a shift away from an emphasis on 'inspection' to health promotion (Box 5.1).

Despite considerable variation across the country in the content and organization of health services for school-age children, the Department of Health argues that there is a consensus emerging among health authorities for a more selective approach concentrating on seven key functions (Box 5.2).

In the context of these objectives, whilst recognizing that legislation does not require a health service *in school* – for instance, children could be 'inspected' in a primary-care setting – the Department of Health envisages a 'continuing and evolving' role for a school health service. It also agrees with the British Paediatric Association (1995) that school settings provide appropriately child-centred and educational environments for this work (Department of Health 1996, para 8.4).

Box 5.1 Objectives of the school health service

◆ Supporting teachers and parents in the delivery of health education.

◆ Providing health advice to children and to those with responsibility for the education and welfare of school children.

◆ Encouraging and enabling children to take responsibility for their own health and well-being, thereby preparing them to be the parents of the future.

◆ Minimizing the consequences of illness and disability in children for their education.

◆ Reducing preventable causes of ill health, impairment and disability. (Department of Health 1996, para 8.2)

Box 5.2 Key functions of the school health service

◆ Complementing primary care services by providing a 'safety net' for children who may not have received a full programme of child health surveillance before starting school.

◆ Monitoring completeness of immunization and providing selected immunizations.

◆ Health advice to school staff, parents and children.

◆ Identification of social care needs including need for protection from abuse.

◆ Aiding liaison between schools, primary care teams, social services departments and secondary care services in meeting the health and social care needs of children.

◆ Identification of special educational needs – a health service contribution to the assessment and support of children with special educational needs and medical problems, in both special and mainstream schools.

◆ Health promotion – support to teachers in the delivery of health education and other health-promoting activities informed by the government's Health of the Nation health-promoting strategy and reinforced by the Health of the Young Nation initiative.
(Department of Health 1996, para 8.6)

School nursing

School nurses comprise the only branch of the profession with specific responsibilities for the school-age group. However, since the workforce is small, nurses carry large caseloads. According to a recent survey carried out by the Health Visitors' Association, the average caseload is just over 2000 school children, although this figure masks considerable variation (Health Visitors' Association 1996). Historically, with a focus on medical inspection, the service has been led by school doctors, with nurses in a supporting role. However, as long as 20 years ago, in its landmark review of child health services, the Court Report acknowledged opportunities for school nursing, urging that nurses be seen as 'the representatives of health in the everyday life of the school' (Department of Health and Social Security 1976, para 10.13).

In recent years, with more emphasis within the service on health promotion, the respective roles of doctor and nurse have changed. Medical examinations are now typically carried out on a selective basis, following a health assessment by the nurse, with school doctors tending to focus on children with special needs. The school nurse is now widely acknowledged as the lead health professional in school, acting as 'the main focus point for the whole school population' (British Paediatric Association 1995, p. viii).

Much of the time of school nurses is still taken up with routine school child health surveillance, comprising periodic measurements of height and weight, along with screening tests to check vision and hearing. Many school nurses also carry out immunization programmes in schools. The content and timing of this work vary across the country since it is determined locally through service contracts negotiated between individual NHS trusts and health commissioners.

Apart from this work, the role of the school nurse is typically not prescribed. Our own research found considerable variation in activities among school nurses. However, we were able to identify four key roles of the school nurse:

◆ assessing the health of children
◆ promoting health
◆ acting as a confidante for children and young people
◆ supporting families.

An overarching role of the school nurse was that of health adviser, not only to school-age children but also to parents and teachers. This work also included liaison with other professionals in education, health and social care services. The empirical part of the chapter provides evidence of ways in which school nurses are interpreting their role in practice.

POLICY CONTEXT

So far, we have set out background information to the current role of school nursing services and drawn attention to guidance from the Department of Health suggesting how it sees this role developing. We now move on to discuss three broad policy themes with particular importance for school nursing: a focus on a needs-led service; an emphasis on health promotion; and a shift from secondary to primary care. Later sections of the chapter use our empirical findings to consider the implications of these policy developments for school nursing.

A needs-led service

There are two linked aspects of the current policy trend of needs-led services which have significance for school nursing. First, the general requirement to deliver services on the basis of assessed need. Second, policy developments encourage agencies and professionals to pay more attention to listening and responding to need as expressed by users themselves.

Assessing needs

The NHS and Community Care Act 1990 confirmed the commitment of the NHS to provide services based on needs. Such a commitment should be a boost to school nurses, whose work centres on assessing the health of the school-age population and seeking to respond to identified needs. Yet despite this potential contribution to a major objective of health policy, some NHS trusts across the country are reducing their investment in school nursing services. In their recent study, DeBell & Everett (1997) found no evidence that decisions to disinvest in school nursing had been informed by any systematic service evaluation and they argue that the relative invisibility of the school nursing service may be part of the problem. Our own research suggests that commissioners have poor understanding of the role of the school nurse. Moreover, since services for school-age children are subject to few statutory requirements and little national guidance, they argue that this client group is inevitably given low priority.

> *Until someone makes school-age children a national priority they are going to come a bit further down the ladder.* (Health commissioner)

Accordingly, commissioners in our study have not pursued systematic assessment of the health needs of their local school-age populations, which might include synthesizing data collected routinely by school nurses.

It is nevertheless widely acknowledged that the health needs of children have changed since the school medical service was set up at the turn of the century. Certainly, the major threats to the survival of children which prompted its development have receded, largely through public health measures such as improved sanitation, housing and immunizations (McKeown 1979). However, as Woodroffe et al report in their 1993 review of available data on child health, new concerns have arisen such as emotional and behavioural difficulties, unhealthy lifestyles and protecting children from harm, along with the need to support the increasing numbers of children who now survive with chronic illness and disabilities. However, without systematic assessment of local health needs, it is difficult for commissioners and service managers to be clear about the overall direction and priorities of services for children which would, in turn, provide a framework for the professional role of nursing. A national survey of NHS trusts in England providing school health services found that one-third had no strategy for the service (Bagnall & Dilloway 1996a).

The lack of a clear strategic remit for school nursing allows for significant variations in practice between nurses. Whilst it might be argued that nurses are best placed to identify and respond to local needs, lack of consensus among nurses about their role – and a corresponding lack of clear understanding on the part of colleagues and users – brings with it a number of problems for nurses in realizing their potential, as will become apparent throughout this chapter. Findings from the research suggest that contracts for school health work are still largely characterized by a historical preoccupation with health surveillance and screening of the school population. However, reappraisal of the role of the welfare state at national policy level favours a shift to delivering services on a selective basis. Such a shift represents a considerable challenge to the traditional universalist model adopted by school health. Taking decisions about how best to target professional efforts is particularly difficult for a service which receives little national policy attention, is not steered by guidance on priorities and has developed little work on the effectiveness of existing interventions in meeting needs. Given limited resources, together with the changing health needs of school-age children, there is an urgent requirement to evaluate the effectiveness of current health services for this client group, including the scope for a more selective focus, based on need.

Involving service users

User involvement has been a cornerstone of health and welfare policy in the 1990s and is designed to improve services through agencies and professionals responding to needs expressed by users themselves. Such a movement is closely linked to notions about the rights of users, about which propositions have flourished in various welfare sectors in the form of 'charters' (for example, Department of Health 1991, Department for Education and Employment 1996). Although these developments appear to have been made typically with adults in mind, there has also been a parallel movement to promote the rights of children. The Children Act 1989, in unifying much of the existing legislation about children, established three important principles underpinning service provision:

◆ reinforcing the position of parents as holding primary responsibility for their children, with services in a supporting role, acting in 'partnership' with families;
◆ establishing that, in all decisions affecting the child, his or her welfare is paramount;
◆ acknowledging the rights of the child to have a voice in such decisions.

The United Nations Convention on the Rights of the Child, to which the UK is a signatory, stresses the rights of children to special consideration as particularly vulnerable members of society, including their rights to health (United Nations 1992). As in the Children Act 1989, the rights of children to have their views heard and respected is paramount. In the UK, the Patient's Charter: Services for Children and Young People establishes rights of access to child health care, with specific commitments made in respect of health visitors and school nurses (NHS Executive 1996a). Although responsibility for children's health is usually assumed by families – particularly for young children

– developments to promote the rights of children have implications for the way in which services are provided and so for the professionals who deliver them.

Involving children as service users has particular relevance for young people since, as children grow older, they increasingly take responsibility for their own health (Brannen et al 1994, Mayall 1994). However, in their routine encounters with health services, children are likely to be accompanied by a parent or another adult, so in practice they may have few opportunities to express their own views as service users. It follows that independent contact with a nurse, in the familiar environment of school, may be one of the few means children have to talk to a health professional in confidence. In seeking to respond to the views of users, professionals must be clear about exactly who the users of their services are. Although the work of school nurses focuses on children, there are other users, in particular parents and school staff. Tensions can exist for nurses, both in attempting to meet the needs of all users and in reconciling their differing views as to what constitutes an appropriate nursing role for children. School nurses are at the forefront of dealing with the particularly complicated issue of balancing the needs and wishes of adult carers with those of children themselves.

Promoting health

In recent years, there have been moves to shift the focus in health work away from reliance on the narrow 'biomedical' view of health as the absence of disease towards a wider definition strengthening health promotion and the prevention of ill health (World Health Organization 1985). In 1992, the government published Health of the Nation, a strategy document including targets for improved health status in England in five key areas: coronary heart disease and stroke; cancers; mental illness; HIV/AIDS and sexual health; and accidents (Department of Health 1992). Although only two of the five areas include targets specifically for children and young people – conceptions under 16 years and childhood accidents – the theme for the third year (1995) of this key policy was the Health of the Young Nation, acknowledging the importance of working with young people in improving the nation's health (Department of Health 1995a). Working with a captive audience in the educational and everyday setting of schools, school nurses are potentially ideally placed to make a contribution to young people's health (British Paediatric Association 1995). However, school nurses have no mandate to carry out health promotion work in school. For example, under the Education Act 1993, it is schools who have formal responsibilities for health education. In seeking to develop this aspect of their work, school nurses must negotiate their role with staff in individual schools, with the prospect of varying degrees of success.

A primary care-led NHS

The major shift in emphasis from secondary to primary care heralded by the NHS and Community Care Act 1990 has brought the work of community-based nurses into sharper policy and managerial focus (NHS Management Executive 1993, Department of Health/NHS Management Executive 1993). Within this shift, general practice is seen as playing a pivotal role, both as commissioner of local services and as an organizational basis for service provision (NHS Management Executive 1993). A focus on the services of GPs and their general practice-based colleagues inevitably risks marginalizing community health services such as school health which are less easily appropriately delivered according to this model. At one level there are practical problems of 'attaching' school nurses to local practices. At a more fundamental level, the shift to a primary care-led NHS raises questions about the continued value of population-based, community health services, such as school health.

At the same time, however, two policy developments offer new prospects for integrating better the work with children carried out by different nurses in a variety of settings, such as GP surgeries, clinics, family homes and schools. The first of these developments is 'locality commissioning', through which GPs can have purchasing power over services such as school health (NHS Executive 1995a, King's Fund 1997). Secondly, following a White Paper on the future of primary care (NHS Executive 1996b), under the NHS (Primary Care) Act 1997 there is a strong commitment to develop new partnership models of working, including those led by nurses.

POLICY DEVELOPMENTS AND THE ROLE OF THE SCHOOL NURSE

How do school nurses work in ways consistent with current policy aspirations? What are the constraints in developing their role and reaching their potential? And how might these be overcome? In this section, we consider the implications of the three policy themes discussed above – a focus on needs-led services; an emphasis on health promotion; and a shift in favour of primary health care – for the role of school nursing. To do this, we move on from policy analysis to address key empirical questions about the contribution of school nursing to child health and the challenges to its developing role. We do so by drawing on research evidence from our study of school nursing.

A needs-led service

Assessing the health needs of individual children

School nursing has the lead role in assessing the health of individual school-age children. Each NHS trust with school health services operates its own surveillance programmes: those in our four study sites differed from each other in both timing and content. In all the sites school nurses used 'health-care interviews' to assess the health of new school entrants. Although these interviews usually incorporated traditional screening for vision and hearing and monitoring of growth and development, nurses believed that health-care interviews enabled them to take a more holistic approach to health assessment. Parents were usually invited to interviews for new entrants, providing an opportunity to discuss any health concerns about their children.

In addition to formal arrangements for school child health surveillance, school nurses also have informal opportunities to find out about children's health needs; in particular, talking to teachers may reveal health-related concerns about individual pupils. Their more regular contact with the same groups of children generally places teachers in a better position than nurses to spot any health problems. However, our study revealed that the school nurse was seen by teachers as someone with special expertise in health and who, unlike teachers, is free from obligations to the rest of the class and so able to focus on the needs of individual children.

Assessing the health needs of school populations

Since the school nurse caseload comprises the pupil rolls of a number of schools, it follows that these nurses are uniquely placed among health professionals to develop health-needs assessment work at local school population level. In doing so, school nurses not only have opportunities for targeting their own work, but also for establishing a knowledge base relating to the public health objectives of commissioning (Department of Health 1995b,c). However, our research found this aspect of health-needs assessment underdeveloped among practitioners. Only one of our study sites had developed a systematic approach to school-health profiling. Evidence from these profiles was used as a means of targeting the work of nurses both within and between schools. Elsewhere, experience of profiling was limited to 'one-off' exercises as part of school-nurse training. Although generally in favour of profiling in principle, nurses cited lack of time as the reason for not developing this aspect of their work. These nurses allocated any remaining time after the completion of surveillance work according to their 'best guess' judgements about the needs of individual schools.

Involving service users

School nurses can offer opportunities for young people to talk to a health professional independently in the familiar setting of school, either at the school entry health-care interview, at 'drop-ins' or in passing in the school corridor or playground. Where nurses in our study sites were offering a health-care interview for secondary school pupils, nurses preferred parents not to be present so that young people could talk themselves, in keeping with policy trends to encourage young people to take control of their own health. There was some evidence that nurses were attempting to use the information collected in these sessions to influence the type of health information available in schools.

Although young people told us they were most likely to turn first to other family members or a teacher with their health concerns, an important role for the school nurse emerged as a trusted alternative adult when neither parent or teacher is appropriate. One parent of a child in high school remarked:

> *The school nurse offers a link for a child who's got worries. Perhaps they can't go to their parent. They know there's someone approachable that they can go to who isn't a teacher – some children don't like to go to teachers.*

In response to these needs and to create opportunities for self-referral, many nurses in the study were running 'drop-in' sessions for children and young people to talk with a nurse in confidence at school.

In seeking to take an holistic approach, school nurses work with pupils not only directly but also indirectly, through supporting adults who care for children, in particular parents and teachers.

> *It's not just looking at the child, it's looking at the child within the family setting as well as the school setting.* (School nurse)

Some school nurses were running 'drop-in' advice sessions for parents in primary schools in response to their knowledge that parents valued the skills of nurses in listening to and advising on what parents deemed 'niggly' health worries about their children. Examples of support given to families by school nurses included practical help, such as liaising with social services departments, and emotional support for parents in coping with children with behaviour problems and other family difficulties.

Perceiving children as users of services, however, highlights tensions for nurses where children and young people, parents and school staff may have differing views as to the health needs of school-age children. In short, an important influence on school nursing work is the extent to which it is mediated by other adult 'gatekeepers'. Parents can act as gatekeepers by withdrawing their children from certain sessions, for instance, sex education. Further, although 'drop-in' sessions for pupils were common in the secondary schools in our study, nurses were reluctant to consider working in this way in primary schools where children's health was judged to be more legitimately under parental control. However, the key gatekeepers to emerge from our research were school governors and staff. Since schools are only formally required to facilitate routine child health surveillance and immunization programmes, nurses must negotiate any additional work with staff in each school. As a result, school staff influence the content and frequency of encounters between nurses and pupils, together with the working conditions in which these encounters take place.

Poor working conditions are thought to limit the potential for school health work (Henshelwood & Polnay 1994). In our own study, nurses and young people drew attention to a lack of privacy for drop-in sessions, together with problems securing anonymity, particularly where the room used was in a prominent location, for instance, next to the head's office or the canteen or on a main thoroughfare within the building.

> *It's private inside, she (the school nurse) never tells anyone what you're talking about, but it's not private because everyone knows you've been in there.* (Girl aged 13)

Despite the implications for service access and take-up by children arising from the 'gatekeeping' activities of schools, this role appeared to be accepted by nurses and their managers as part of embedded practice. Nurses talked about having so-called 'difficult' schools on their caseload where they were allowed insufficient or no access to pupils beyond health surveillance and immunization activities. Reluctantly, attempts to negotiate access might have to be abandoned, despite a nurse's view as to the consequences for unmet need. Some head teachers held strong views as to their position as users of school nursing services. They drew attention to confusion about the role of the nurse and to a corresponding need for closer liaison with school health managers to secure a framework for understanding their service entitlement:

> *We haven't got a clue what's on offer ... we don't know what her (the school nurse's) position is at all, if she can deliver what she's interested in, or whether she should be. It needs to be (looked at) beyond the people on the ground. Health should say what's on offer and see if that's what schools want or whether other things are more important. We're the customer in effect, but no-one is saying is this what you want?* (Head, middle school)

In seeking to raise awareness about the potential role of the nurse in school and to reconcile differences in views about health needs between nurses and school staff, our research did find support for some kind of framework, or 'service level agreement', between individual schools and the local NHS trust for school health services. Pilot work for the Department of Health has suggested that such an approach can also deliver a number of other benefits (Box 5.3).

An important question is who should determine the health needs of school-age children. While service level agreements can help arbitrate between the perspectives of adults, incorporating the views of children and young people themselves more systematically seems likely to bring the best prospects for matching services most closely to their needs as ultimate users.

> **Box 5.3** Negotiating school health services
>
> Service level agreements between schools and their local NHS trusts can
> help to:
> ◆ raise the profile of the school nurse;
> ◆ encourage a proactive response to needs;
> ◆ draw together health and education priorities to determine health targets
>   jointly;
> ◆ plan jointly for health promotion;
> ◆ plan health surveillance so as to minimize disruption in school;
> ◆ improve working relationships;
> ◆ provide better information than in exisiting contracts for NHS
>   commissioning purposes.
>
> (Department of Health 1994)

The potential of school nursing

In the context of a policy focus on needs-led services, school nurses are arguably well placed to play a central role. However, they are currently thwarted
in doing so by a number of factors. One difficulty is that of time. School nurses
carry large caseloads and work under severe time constraints. Although they
are potentially well placed to develop the relationships which are important
for children for expressing their needs, in practice this appears difficult for
nurses to achieve and so many needs are likely to remain hidden. Further, the
requirement to assess the needs of individual children – in particular through
formal surveillance programmes – inevitably places a lower priority on
population-level work, despite its potential benefits.

Second, in the absence of a 'blueprint' for the school health service (Bagnall
& Dilloway 1996a), practice varies a good deal, not only between NHS trusts
but also between individual nurses. Although this situation allows potential
for nurses to develop the services they offer in response to needs, it risks
poor understanding of their role by school staff, which is crucial for a service
requiring mediation by 'gatekeeping' schools. A strategic framework could
lead to more effective targeting of school nursing resources through focusing
nursing activities and securing improved support from managers.

Third, our research found few connections linking the activities of practitioners and commissioners. To the observer, it is a curious paradox that
health-needs assessment of school-age children should remain underdeveloped when, at the same time, services are commissioned which employ a
group of professionals charged with finding out the health needs of children.

Data collected by nurses do not appear to be aggregated or manipulated for commissioning purposes. The lack of computerized information systems was frequently cited by nurses as preventing the data from being used more extensively. Conversely, school nurses do not appear to have access to local epidemiological information, which is available to commissioners, to help target their practice.

Health promotion

The role of the school nurse

Increased emphasis on health promotion within health policy is central to current developments in the role of school nursing. In our study, the impact of the Health of the Nation was clear, nurses consistently citing it as steering their work, both in respect of specific targets – such as teenage conception rates – and the importance of promoting healthy lifestyles among children and young people (Department of Health 1992). Although the bulk of their time is spent on health assessments of individual pupils, our research found strong, although not universal, support from school nurses for a shift in favour of greater involvement in health promotion. Some school nurses argued that routine health surveillance might be delegated to support nurses to free more (qualified) school nursing time, enabling them to respond to other needs. Skill mix within teams of school nurses was being used in one of the study sites in order to make more effective use of differing skills.

School nurses commonly identified classroom work as an area they wished to develop. Existing contributions included providing information and materials for teachers and direct involvement in lessons, with or without a teacher present. School nurses were also sometimes involved in wider school health promotion activities, such as 'health weeks'.

Despite school nurses being well placed to promote health among school-age children, developing such a role presents a number of challenges. First, since health education is a crosscurricular theme, there is scope for considerable variation between schools in the level of priority and time given by teachers both to classroom health education and other ways of promoting health. It follows that staff in some schools are more interested than those in others to explore the potential contribution of the school nurse.

A second issue in developing this aspect of school nursing work concerns differentiating the nursing role from that of others in health promotion. For instance, within the NHS there is a network of health promotion officers, some of whom provide advice to schools, and in schools, teachers have formal responsibility for health education. It follows that nurses must be clear about the distinctiveness and value of their contribution. Probing in some depth the role of the school nurse as a teacher of sex education, our study found that the distinctive nursing contribution had five linked aspects:

- expert and up-to-date knowledge;
- an informal style, conducive to discussion on sensitive topics;
- comfortable when talking about the body;
- a non-judgemental approach
- being an 'outsider' to whom young people can put questions on sensitive or controversial matters without fear of repercussions in school:

> *They (nurses) bring a dimension which is so different from teachers ... it's difficult to describe but ... they're unmoralizing, unshockable and not perceived by children as having moral authority over them.* (Deputy head, high school)

Although many school nurses felt passionately that a teaching role should be central to the development of school nursing, there was no universal consensus among the nurses in the study. Crucially, while some school nurses have taken postregistration courses in health education or teaching, these skills do not comprise a core component of nurse education itself. Guarding against the risks of nurses being deployed as surrogate teachers, the Department of Health has declared that it 'does not consider that nurses should "teach" classes on their own' (Department of Health 1996, para 8.10).

The potential for school nursing

Our evidence suggests that there are at least two areas in which the role of the school nurse might be further developed in respect of health promotion: the first is that of mental health and the second relates to achieving a 'balance' between the elements of health promotion. Although Woodroffe et al (1993) observed that there is little information available nationally on mental ill health among young people, there has been growing concern about the likely extent of these needs coupled with a lack of existing services. In our study, school nurses faced something of an impasse, aware of both limited opportunities for referring young people to appropriate services and the need to draw careful boundaries in terms of their own counselling abilities. Some school nurses were responding directly to mental health promotion needs. For instance, profiling the health of a secondary school population, a school nurse realized that there had been four attempted suicides among pupils. Together with a teacher, she set up sessions within the personal and social education programme to promote self-esteem. As a 'first-tier' service, the role of the school nurse in promoting mental health is consistent with recommendations of the recent major review of child and adolescent mental health services (NHS Health Advisory Service 1995).

Our second suggestion concerns the appropriate balance of activity within health promotion work and stems from the views of young people about their health. In our discussions, young people revealed a keen awareness of the structural factors influencing health, such as low income and poor housing. This evidence suggests that existing individualistic approaches to health promotion, such as health education, may have limited impact and might be balanced by a wider public health approach. Although our research revealed examples of innovative work of this type, it appears that the potential for school nurses to work in this way is underexploited.

A primary care-led NHS

Although nursing services dedicated to school-age children are provided by school nurses, largely but not exclusively in schools, a range of other nurses may work with school-age children. This work takes place in a variety of settings, including GP surgeries as part of PHCTs and in community health clinics. It was clear from our study that health commissioners, service managers and practitioners are beginning to question the continuing role of the school health service in the light of a policy emphasis which has at its core a primary care-led NHS. At the heart of these deliberations are issues concerning appropriate models and settings for nursing work with children and how best to integrate the work of different nurses in order to make the best use of resources in meeting needs. While our study focused on the existing roles of the school nurse, analysis of the findings brings evidence to bear on two key questions: how appropriate is school as a setting for nursing work and what are the possible ways of integrating nursing support for all school-age children?

School as a setting for nursing work

The research suggests there are both advantages and disadvantages associated with school-based nursing work (Box 5.4). Despite these considerable advantages, there are also some disadvantages (Box 5.5).

Box 5.4 Advantages of school as a setting for nursing work

- ◆ A 'captive' population for efficient delivery of health surveillance and screening programmes.
- ◆ A 'child-centred' and 'educational' environment, facilitating health promotion work.
- ◆ The nurse can act as a bridge between the health and education systems.
- ◆ The nurse offers an on-site opportunity for young people to seek confidential health advice independently.
- ◆ Working at school population level offers potential for the school nurse to profile health needs and influence school policies.

> **Box 5.5** The disadvantages associated with school as a setting for nursing work
>
> ◆ The 'gatekeeping' role of schools influences variation in access to and take-up of nursing services by pupils.
> ◆ Working in a non-NHS setting can lead to isolation from NHS colleagues, inhibiting collaboration.
> ◆ The caseload of the school nurse typically appears to extend only to children on school rolls. It is unclear how children not attending school obtain support in meeting their health needs.
> ◆ Not all young people wish to take up services based in school premises. A choice of access points to service support is valued by young people.

Overall, our research findings support the case for a nursing role in school. Most children attend school and the study evidence suggests that health-related support is an expected and acceptable part of everyday school life which is also easy to access. Searching out health needs and the capacity to adopt a community, in addition to an individualistic, focus are features of school health work which have not hitherto characterized work in general practice. However, the disadvantages associated with working in a school setting point to a need to consider not only how nursing can maximize its potential in schools but, perhaps more fundamentally, also how nursing can make an appropriate contribution to meeting the needs of all school-age children, in and out of school.

Potential for integrating school nursing and PHCT nursing services

Our research found the drive for a primary care-led NHS is providing new motivation for managers and professionals to think about closer integration between the work of PHCTs and school health services. However, considerable problems were reported in achieving this goal. Given the small number of school nurses, together with the mismatch between GP practices and school populations, 'attaching' school nurses to general practice in the same way as for district nurses and health visitors is not regarded as feasible. Furthermore, on the whole school nurses reported that collaboration with colleagues in PHCTs was weak and their role poorly understood, particularly by GPs. Although some radical ideas were aired in the study – for instance, developing 'integrated nursing teams' of practice nurses, health visitors and school nurses – in practice the emphasis was on how school nurses might be more closely 'aligned' with PHCTs.

EDUCATION AND PREPARATION OF SCHOOL NURSES

Historically, school nurses have achieved lower professional status than other community health nurses. There is no mandatory specialist qualification required to practise as a school nurse unlike, for example, a health visitor. However, fundamental changes in nurse education at both pre- and post-registration levels are affecting how nurses are prepared to care for school children's health.

Preregistration level

The route into school nursing for the majority of school nurses has been the traditional registered general nurse (RGN) qualification, which has predominantly focused on the care of adults. Although registered sick children's nurses (RSCNs) have been able to enter school nursing, the focus of this preparation has been on the care of sick children in hospital. Moreover, as the Health Visitors Association found in its recent survey, only 12% of school nurses are qualified as RSCNs (Health Visitors' Association 1996).

Developments in nurse education mean that the RSCN qualification is being phased out in favour of the Project 2000 registered nurse (child branch) diploma. This course allows students to specialize in child health at preregistration level. In placing equal emphasis on health and ill health, the course also allows students to gain experience in a variety of community settings, including schools, in addition to hospital care. The impact of this new qualification on the skills and competencies of those entering school nursing has yet to be evaluated. However, it seems likely that the equal emphasis placed on health and illness in Project 2000 programmes will prepare child branch nurses better than did traditional forms of preparation to meet the modern-day health needs of school-age children.

Postregistration level

There are no mandatory postregistration requirements to practise as a school nurse. However, the recent HVA survey found that over 50% of school nurses held the School Nurse Certificate (Health Visitors' Association 1996), indicating a desire to acquire additional skills relevant to meeting the health needs of school-age children. The certificate had been awarded following a 12-week course focusing on health monitoring and promotion, but is currently being phased out following implementation of the UKCC's postregistration education and practice reforms (UKCC 1994). Under these reforms, school nursing has become a degree-level qualification. A nurse graduating from this programme will be recorded on the UKCC register as a community health nurse (school nursing) and for the first time will enjoy equal professional status with colleagues in other community health nursing disciplines.

There are fundamental changes in the education and preparation of nurses working with school-age children at both pre- and postregistration levels. The key question relating to these changes is whether nurses working with children should possess specialist skills. Following its recent deliberations on health services for children, the House of Commons Health Committee recommended that the Department of Health 'commit itself to the principle that all nurses for whom children comprise the focus of their work should be qualified children's nurses' (House of Commons Health Committee 1997, para 130). In the light of this recommendation it may be that trusts will turn increasingly to child branch nurses for work with school children and, resources permitting, to developing the knowledge base of existing school nurses through the specialist community practitioner programme.

The developing role of school nursing

Earlier in the chapter we drew attention to wide variations in practice between school nurses and the absence of a strategic framework clarifying their role. Other commentators have also been surprised by the absence of a definitive description of the role (Strehlow 1987), an omission which is increasingly curious given the acknowledged position of the nurse as the lead health professional in school (British Paediatric Association 1995). Whilst there is no clear national remit for school nursing, policy developments described in this chapter have implications for the developing role of school nurses and so for their preparation to practise.

First, the emphasis on health promotion within health policy would suggest a clear role for school nurses in a national health promotion strategy. In practice, however, despite children and young people being widely regarded as a key group for targeting such work, the health promotion role of school nurses appears to be ambiguous and contested. Indeed, the Department of Health appears reluctant to identify health promotion as a role for school nurses, arguing that it has not been central to school nurse education. The appropriate contribution of school nurses to meeting the health promotion needs of children and young people is in urgent need of debate.

The second key implication of policy developments for the role of school nursing relates to needs assessment, particularly in the absence of needs assessment by health commissioners. It might be argued that school nurses, who work closely with children, are ideally placed to identify and respond to the varying health needs of school-age children. Both commissioners and nurses have yet to maximize the potential of information collected routinely by school nurses, let alone the possible benefits for a strategic framework which could arise from systematic profiling of local population needs.

In terms of responding to needs, as accountable professionals, nurses are guided by the Scope of Professional Practice (UKCC 1992), which enables nurses to respond innovatively to need providing they have the necessary knowledge, skills and competencies. However, the lack of a strategic framework for the school nurse role creates difficulties for those responsible for ensuring that core elements of educational programmes reflect the contemporary needs of school-age children. Common examples cited by nurses in the study of developing their role in response to needs included asthma management, counselling and teaching. Despite the high level of need apparent among the school-age population, nurses saw existing school nursing preparation arrangements as inadequate in these fields. In contrast, other aspects of education and training had little in the way of mass application in practice, despite their potential benefits – for example, profiling at school population level.

The potential benefits of a high level of professional autonomy inevitably need to be balanced against the value of regarding the remit of the school nurse. In terms of education, the poorly defined role for school nurses risks mismatching course components with actual needs. Furthermore, clarity of role is crucial at a time of unprecedented questioning of the value of existing services within the NHS. All professionals need skills in marketing their contribution; perhaps particularly so in multiprofessional (and occasionally competitive) fields such as child health.

EVALUATING SCHOOL NURSING SERVICES

Evidence-based practice

The importance of demonstrating effectiveness has grown with the firm commitment made by the NHS to evidence-based practice (see Chapter 10). However, this approach presupposes that sufficient research evidence is available to help practitioners make decisions about effectiveness. As Hicks argues, 'It is axiomatic that clinical practice cannot be informed by research if that research is not published' (Hicks 1996). The paucity of research evidence concerning school nursing is a major stumbling block, not only for nurses wanting to improve their practice but also in demonstrating the effectiveness of services to those responsible for commissioning services.

As accountable professionals, nurses are under increasing pressure to demonstrate the value of their contribution to meeting local health needs. However, evidence from our own study suggests that school nursing services are commissioned largely on an historical basis rather than as any systematic attempt at evaluation. While commissioning on this basis in our study sites was attributed to the low priority attached to school health services, in other parts of the country it appears that a lack of evidence on effectiveness has made school health an easy target for cost-cutting programmes (DeBell & Everett 1997).

Difficulties in evaluating school nursing services

None of our four research sites had measures in place for evaluating school nursing services. Why should this be so? Apart from the low priority given to school health, progress appears to have been hampered by a number of other factors. At a practical level, information systems focusing on counting client 'contacts' for contracting purposes yield few data on outcomes or the quality of nursing interventions. Furthermore, some school nurse interventions are poorly captured by activity recording systems. As a result, these activities remain largely hidden from commissioners and risk being undervalued. For example, one school nurse expressed particular frustration that there was no place to record her drop-in session work on the standard form for recording activities. She had to classify it as 'hygiene', which meant that not only did it remain hidden but this also reinforced assumptions that her work centred on a narrow, physical or 'medical' model of health.

Establishing the effectiveness of school nursing presents further difficulties by the very nature of the work involved: illness prevention and health promotion both suffer from a lack of consensus as to what works when (Lightfoot 1994). In addition, particularly in the case of health promotion, attributing outcomes to particular interventions can be difficult. For example, whilst several school nurses felt their increased involvement with young people on sexual health promotion in schools had helped to reduce the local teenage conception rate, it was impossible to prove or measure the association.

Possible beginnings

One way forward for evaluating school nursing services might be to begin with routine school child health surveillance. Not only does this work comprise a core activity of the service, taking up much of the time of nurses, the nature of this work is amenable to conventional outcome measures, for instance detection of health problems. Another reason for beginning with this work is evidence of the wide variation between NHS trusts in the content and timing of their surveillance interventions, suggesting that there may be some scope to align practices more closely with known effectiveness. Although the relative benefits of different approaches to surveillance are always likely to be contested, the recent report of the BPA includes a suggested core surveillance programme on the evidence available to date (British Paediatric Association 1995). A further benefit of a rigorous examination of health surveillance work is to establish whether resources released from any relaxation of the programme might allow school nurses to use their time more effectively by developing other aspects of their role. Whatever the value of surveillance, school nurses in our study were frustrated at its dominance within their work, arguing that their time might be better used in other ways, for example in meeting emotional health needs.

Of course, the wide variety of other work carried out by school nurses also warrants evaluation. School nurses in the case study sites were beginning to introduce new practices in response to needs expressed by school-age children, but there appeared to be few, if any, signs that these developments were being implemented on the basis of any evidence of effectiveness. Overall, while there is widespread recognition of the need for evaluation – and some local work is beginning to be published (for example, Bagnall & Dilloway 1996b) – there would still appear to be a long way to go in establishing (much-needed) evidence-based practice in school nursing.

Involving service users

Any service evaluation should take account of the views of users, since it is their needs that services are aiming to meet. While some school nurses in our study evaluated their classroom health education work routinely at the end of each session, this is inevitably a short-term measure of effectiveness in meeting needs. However, giving pupils an opportunity to suggest how future sessions might be improved might prompt incremental changes sensitive to users' needs and preferences. Despite exhortation to involve users in the planning and evaluation of services (NHS Management Executive 1992, NHS Executive 1995b), this approach does not seem well developed for children. For instance, the young people in our study had strong views about their service preferences, together with some very practical and modest suggestions for raising awareness of the school nurse, but appeared to have no means of expressing these views.

Overall, it appears that school-age children have limited opportunities to influence services. For instance, the Patient's Charter: Services for Children and Young People couches references to school nursing in terms of what parents can expect for their children rather than in terms of children's rights (NHS Executive 1996a). Furthermore, service entitlement in the Charter is restricted to health surveillance and does not extend to activity which can be steered more easily by users, such as drop-in sessions. Commissioners acknowledged that they did not listen systematically to this group. Yet our discussions with young people suggested that they do have very clear service preferences, such as: privacy; confidentiality; a choice of setting; and services designed for their age group.

Evaluating school nursing in context

School nurses are part of a complex pattern of child health services. As the shift to a primary care-led NHS has helped to make clear, there is a need to evaluate services for children and their families 'in the round', not only on a service-by-service basis. The recent report from the House of Commons Health Committee on health services for children and young people considered a wide variety of nurses with differing specialisms who work with children and urged greater coordination between them (House of Commons Health Committee 1997). One example from our own research concerns health visitors and school nurses. The health visitor typically 'hands over' children on their caseload to the school nurse when they start school, yet parents said they would welcome ongoing contact with their family health visitor. Although we found that some school nurses carry out home visits to provide family support, constraints of time and training limit their capacity to undertake the family visitor role. It follows that the time of starting school, while convenient for demarcating responsibilities between different professionals, does not necessarily meet the needs of families.

CONCLUSION

We set out in this chapter to use our empirical research evidence to examine the current role of school nursing and its potential in the context of three key policy developments: a focus on needs-led services; an emphasis on health promotion; and the shift in favour of a primary care-led NHS. It is impossible to draw firm conclusions in terms of measuring the contribution of school nursing to these policy aspirations: as we have seen, not only is the role of school nurses highly individualized, but much of their work is currently hidden and/or not amenable to conventional forms of measurement.

In our own research, we found evidence of school nurses working well within the spirit of these policy goals: identifying and responding to the needs of individuals; profiling the needs of school populations and targeting services accordingly; developing a variety of approaches to health promotion; and seeking to integrate their work with colleagues in PHCTs. A key problem for school nurses is raising awareness of their contribution to child health beyond the traditional system of school child health surveillance. Further, given the lack of a strategic framework for the school nurse role, there is no guarantee that all school nurses are working in ways which maximize their contribution to policy goals in child health. While a high degree of professional autonomy enables nurses to respond innovatively to local needs, such scope must be balanced against the possible benefits of a clearer strategic framework. Benefits include: a better understanding of the school nurse role by all service users, commissioners and professional colleagues; prospects for aligning education and training programmes more closely to core activities; establishing areas for evaluation and standard setting; securing necessary support from managers (for instance, in negotiations to work in schools); and, where appropriate, identifying the support needs of individual practitioners.

Finally, we wish to draw attention to two areas of school nursing practice which seem particularly underdeveloped in terms of working within current policy goals. The first of these is work at the level of the *school population*, for which school nurses are uniquely placed. School health profiling can help both to target their own work and to support commissioning strategies. The second area of underdeveloped work is a thread running through this chapter concerning *children's rights* as service users to express their own views of needs and service preferences. Here again school nurses are uniquely placed, not only to listen to children but also to collate and communicate their opinions to local policy makers.

At the beginning of this chapter we argued that school nursing was an interesting case to explore in relation to policy developments on account of its multifaceted 'invisibility'. Indeed, the picture is one of a service with potential to make a valuable contribution to contemporary policy goals, but which struggles to overcome problems of low priority, poor understanding and low professional status. For school nursing to succeed in its goals – indeed, to remain in existence – a clear role, based on evidence of need and capable of evaluation, must be developed.

QUESTIONS FOR DISCUSSION

◆ How might school nurses influence the commissioning process?

◆ To what extent do school nurses offer a service based upon what children and young people say they need?

◆ What might be an appropriate balance between health surveillance and health promotion in meeting the modern-day needs of school-age children?

◆ Given the contribution of many others to health promotion, how can the skills of school nurses best be utilized to promote health among young people?

◆ Is the shift in favour of a primary care-led NHS an opportunity or a threat for school nursing?

◆ Should school nurses be qualified children's nurses? What might be the advantages and disadvantages?

◆ What information would be needed to evaluate the effectiveness of school nursing work?

ANNOTATED BIBLIOGRAPHY

Woodroffe C, Glickman M, Barker M, Power C 1993 Children, teenagers and health: the key data. Open University Press, Buckingham

A useful book for those who wish to know more about child health statistics so as to consider the likely contemporary health needs of children and young people.

While A E, Barriball K L 1993 School nursing: history, present practice and possibilities reviewed. Journal of Advanced Nursing 18: 1201–1211

A useful paper for anyone wanting to find out in general terms about this branch of the profession. It includes both a historical overview and a discussion of more recent issues and has a useful list of references.

Bagnall P, Dilloway M 1996 In a different light: school nurses and their role in meeting the health needs of school age children. Department of Health/The Queen's Nursing Institute, London

Historically there have been few published empirical studies of school nursing. Recently there has been more activity and this report brings together three local studies on different aspects of school nursing work.

REFERENCES

Bagnall P, Dilloway M 1996a In search of a blueprint: a survey of school health services. Department of Health and The Queen's Nursing Institute, London

Bagnall P, Dilloway M 1996b In a different light: school nurses and their role in meeting the health needs of school age children. Department of Health and The Queen's Nursing Institute, London

Brannen J, Dodd K, Oakley A, Storey P 1994 Young people, health and family life. Open University Press, Buckingham

British Paediatric Association 1995 Health needs of school age children. British Paediatric Association, London

DeBell D, Everett G 1997 In a class apart: a study of school nursing. The Research Centre, City College, Norwich

Department for Education and Employment 1996 Our children's education: the updated parent's charter. Department for Education and Employment, London

Department of Health 1991 The patient's charter. HMSO, London

Department of Health 1992 The health of the nation: a strategy for health in England. Cmnd 1986. HMSO, London

Department of Health 1994 Negotiating school health services. Department of Health, London

Department of Health 1995a Health of the young nation. Unpublished Fact Sheets, July 1995

Department of Health 1995b Making it happen: public health – the contribution, role and development of nurses, midwives and health visitors. Report of the Standing Nursing and Midwifery Advisory Committee. Department of Health, London

Department of Health 1995c Nurses and purchasing. Change, challenge, opportunity: school nurses in the new health service structure. Department of Health, London

Department of Health 1996 Child health in the community: a guide to good practice. NHS Executive, London

Department of Health and Social Security 1976 Fit for the future: report of the committee on child health services. Cmnd 6684 (the Court report). Department of Health and Social Security, London

Department of Health NHS Management Executive 1993 A vision for the future: the nursing, midwifery and health visiting contribution to health and health care. Department of Health, London

Harris B 1995 The health of the schoolchild: a history of the school medical service in England and Wales. Open University Press, Buckingham

Harrison A, Gretton J 1986 School health: the invisible service. In: Harrison A, Gretton J (eds) Health care UK 1986. Policy Journals, London

Health Visitors' Association 1996 School nursing: here today for tomorrow. HVA, London

Henshelwood J, Polnay L J 1994 Facilities for the school health team. Archives of Disease in Childhood 70: 542–544

Hicks C 1996 Nurse researcher: a study of a contradiction in terms? Journal of Advanced Nursing 24: 357–363

House of Commons Health Committee 1997 Third report. Health services for children and young people in the community: home and school. The Stationery Office, London

King's Fund 1997 Total purchasing: a profile of national pilot projects. King's Fund Publishing, London

Lightfoot J 1994 Demonstrating the value of health visiting. Health visitor 67 (1): 19–20

Lightfoot J, Bines W 1997 Keeping children healthy: the role of school nursing. Summary Research Report. Social Policy Research Unit, University of York

Mayall B 1994 Negotiating health: children at home and primary school. Cassell, London

McKeown T 1979 The role of medicine. Basil Blackwell, Oxford

NHS Executive 1995a Developing NHS purchasing and GP fundholding, health service guidelines HSG(85)4. NHS Executive, London

NHS Executive 1995b Priorities and planning guidance for the NHS: 1996/97. NHS Executive, London

NHS Executive 1996a Patient's Charter: services for children and young people. NHS Executive, London

NHS Executive 1996b Primary care: the future. Department of Health, London

NHS Health Advisory Service 1995 Together we stand: the commissioning role and management of child and adolescent mental health services. HMSO, London

NHS Management Executive 1992 Local voices: the views of local people in purchasing for health. NHS Management Executive, London

NHS Management Executive 1993 New world, new opportunities: nursing in primary health care. NHSME, London

Strehlow M 1987 Nursing in educational settings. Lippincott Nursing Series, London

UKCC 1992 The scope of professional practice. UKCC, London

UKCC 1994 The future of professional practice – the council's standards for education and practice following registration. UKCC, London

United Nations 1992 Convention on the rights of the child. Treaty Series 44. HMSO, London

Vine P 1991 Ninety nine and counting. Health visitor 64 (5): 150–151

While A E, Barriball K L 1993 School nursing: history, present practice and possibilities reviewed. Journal of advanced nursing 18: 1201–1211

Woodroffe C, Glickman M, Barker M, Power C 1993 Children, teenagers and health: the key data. Open University Press, Buckingham

World Health Organization 1985 Targets for health for all. WHO Regional Office for Europe, Copenhagen

6

Evaluation and community psychiatric nursing

Peter A. Morrall

KEY ISSUES

- ◆ The role of the community psychiatric nurse is ill defined.
- ◆ Psychiatric nurses working in the community have a significant degree of clinical autonomy.
- ◆ Autonomy in community psychiatric nursing practice must be balanced with the need to ensure rigour in the delivery of mental health services.

INTRODUCTION

This chapter presents empirical evidence from a study of the role, performance and professional status of community psychiatric nurses (CPNs) working in community mental health teams (CMHTs). The focus of the research was directed towards identifying and evaluating the levels of clinical autonomy experienced by psychiatric nurses working in CMHTs.

CLINICAL AUTONOMY

Throughout its history, community psychiatric nursing has tried to produce an identity which is not only separate from nursing generally but is also distinct from 'institutional' mental nursing. This is displayed, for example, in the assertion by CPNs that they function (unlike their hospital counterparts) as autonomous practitioners or have the capacity to do so. An account by Hally of her day's work as a CPN is indicative of how these practitioners have come to regard themselves as 'special'. Making the distinction between community psychiatric nursing and all other areas of nursing, she proclaims that the CPN is:

> ... *a community mental health worker who is an autonomous practitioner*
> ... *there is no other branch of nursing which offers the variety, the challenge, the autonomy and the satisfaction of community psychiatric nursing.*
> (Hally 1989)

For Freidson the main method by which medicine and other professions attain high status is through the acquisition of discrete areas of work and by gaining a socially and legally recognized right to work autonomously. That is, people who are considered to belong to a profession '... have the special privilege of freedom from the control of outsiders' (Freidson 1988). The power of the medical profession depends on a large amount of autonomy over clinical work. In the study reported here, it is Freidson's depiction of professionalism, with his emphasis on the professional being able to determine extensively '... the content and the terms of work' (1970), that is employed to assess the occupational status of CPNs.

RESEARCH AIMS

The study examined the working practices of 10 psychiatric nurses operating as members of four CMHTs in northern England. Apart from the CPNs, the teams consisted of social workers, psychologists, occupational therapists and consultant psychiatrists. The evaluation of the CPNs' levels of clinical autonomy was achieved by monitoring the referral process (and the decision-making processes) from the stage when new clients were referred to the CPN to when they were discharged or re-referred to another health-care professional. Where clients were not discharged or referred (i.e. treatment by the

---

Box 6.1 Community psychiatric nursing: background history

Community psychiatric nursing, a subdivision of mental health nursing, has a relatively short history. But the importance of CPNs in the mental health field leads Armstrong (1987) to claim that they are the '... frontline workers of psychiatric care'.

The community aspect of psychiatric nursing can be traced back to 1954 when two nurses were seconded from a mental hospital in Surrey to work as 'outpatient nurses' because of a shortage of social workers. Their role was to keep contact with discharged patients and to help maintain these patients in the community.

CPN continued), the collection of data stopped after a 3-month period. Questions relevant to these processes include the following.

◆ Does the system of referring clients indicate that the CPNs have clinical autonomy?
◆ Do the CPNs have autonomy over their decisions once a client is referred to them?

The professional status of the CPNs was further assessed by examining the opinions of their colleagues in the CMHTs and the managers to whom the CPNs were directly accountable. Relevant questions on how the CPNs' colleagues and managers view the CPNs include the following.

◆ What are the opinions of the members of the CMHT and the managers about the role, knowledge and skills of the CPN?
◆ Is there any interdisciplinary conflict or hierarchy within the CMHT?

THE CONTEXT OF THE STUDY

As we approach the end of the 20th century, the cultural, economic and technical fabric of 'postindustrial' societies is changing dramatically and unpredictably. For example, the globalization of sophisticated electronic communication systems is creating a new type of social structure which Jones (1995) has termed 'cybersociety'. In cybersociety we find that mass media and computers alter the ways in which we work, conduct our leisure time and interact with each other. Moreover, the computer age has given birth to novel kinds of 'madness' (Morrall 1997a). For example, the Internet has been blamed for creating a form of addiction akin to alcoholism or excessive gambling (Griffiths cited in Ezard 1997) and an epidemic of shyness (Zimbardo cited in Mihill, 1997).

Rapid changes are evident in the systems we use for producing goods and services. Similarly, there are major transformations occurring in the way in which we conceptualize and operate health services. A former Secretary of State for Health commented:

The last decade has seen dramatic changes in the way in which mental health services are organized and, indeed, changes in the whole approach to the concept of mental health itself. (Bottomley, in Department of Health 1994)

However, there is little collective agreement between politicians and leaders of the mental health disciplines. Indeed, the mental health industry can be viewed as being in chaos:

Services for the mentally ill are in turmoil in many parts of Britain ... with

*Government plans setting out how mental patients ought to be cared for ...
being widely ignored.* (Fletcher 1995)

Perhaps the 'chaos' is not surprising when one considers the plethora of
policy initiatives, legislation and recommendations from reports and inquiries
that the mental health services in the United Kingdom have had to face. In the
last few decades, the mental health industry has been required to:

◆ accommodate the independent sector;
◆ disentangle purchasers from providers and health care from social care;
◆ introduce care plans for patients discharged from hospital;
◆ offer non-custodial care and treatment to mentally disordered offenders;
◆ reduce morbidity and suicide rates amongst the mentally ill;
◆ give priority to people placed on supervision registers;
◆ implement a new mental health act;
◆ assess the risk of violence and homicide;
◆ replace care in the community with a 'spectrum' or 'continuum' of care;
◆ prepare for the possibility of an overarching planning and commissioning
  body to 'build bridges' between the various mental health agencies;
◆ respond to the implications of the Patient's Charter;
◆ empower users and carers;
◆ audit clinical practice;
◆ submit mental health practitioners to a series of reviews of their
  practice.

Mental health nursing has always been susceptible to modification due to, for
example, new treatments and changing demands by society (Peplau 1994).
However, the very extent of change occurring in society, the degree of fluctu-
ation in the design and delivery of mental health services and range of policy
initiatives mean that there is little certainty about the direction and role of its
practitioners.

This uncertainty has been recognized in a report from the Sainsbury
Centre for Mental Health which reviewed the roles and training of mental
health staff working in the community (including psychiatric nurses). In this
report, practitioners are viewed as being inadequately prepared for practice.
Furthermore, the report acknowledges much confusion over roles:

*Training and education mechanisms have not moved fast enough to keep
pace with changing service patterns and needs. There are a number of
concerns about the relevance of current training and the fitness to practise of
newly qualified staff. Many staff appear unclear about their roles in a
multi-disciplinary setting and there is a lack of robust mechanisms for
ensuring continuing competent performance after qualifying.*
(Sainsbury Centre 1997)

The lack of clarity of the mental health nurse's role is apparent in a series of policy contradictions. For example, policy makers are demanding that more attention is given to those suffering from 'enduring and serious mental illness', but the health services overall are being guided towards concentrating resources on primary care. Moreover, mental health nurses are caught in a paradox when on the one hand they are encouraged to 'empower' their patients/clients, whilst on the other hand there is pressure for them to 'protect' society from the perceived threat of violence by the mentally disordered. That is, there is little logic for psychiatric nurses to be involved in the promotion of 'mental health' when their role is ultimately one of social control (Morrall, 1998).

The major influence on mental health nursing, however, has been the move from 'asylum' care for the mentally ill to care in the community. Whilst at present only 8% of the 57 000 psychiatric nurses employed in the UK are working in the community, it is predicted that this situation will be reversed in the next few years (Sainsbury Centre 1997). The CMHT is likely to continue to be the most common organizational structure for nurses working outside psychiatric institutions. Therefore, the research study discussed here, in which CPN practice was evaluated in the context of the CMHT, has much relevance to the future shaping of psychiatric nursing in the community.

RESEARCH METHODS

The research strategy had three core components.

◆ A diary-interview schedule formed the core research tool for examining the clinical autonomy and levels of negotiation exercised by the 10 psychiatric nurses. The CMHTs were studied consecutively over a period of 2 years, with the action reportedly taken by the CPNs on 252 new referrals (made to them directly or via the CMHT) being monitored each week. The diary-interview schedule provided a detailed account of the relevant aspects of the CPNs' professional practice and their interpretation of that practice.
◆ Indepth interviewing was used to collect data from the CPNs' colleagues on the CMHT and their managers (as well as being used to complete the diary-interview schedule). Six consultant psychiatrists and five social workers, three psychologists (one of whom represented psychology in two of the CMHTs), four occupational therapists and four nurse managers were interviewed.
◆ Over 150 hours of observation took place during the study. Extended periods of time were spent sitting in the team office or a central area within the team centre.

Following Burgess (1981), substantive observations, preconceptual interpretations of these observations and comments on methodological issues were entered in a field notebook.

The quantitative data from the diary-interview schedule were subjected to statistical analysis using the Statistical Package for the Social Sciences (SPSS/PC-Windows). The procedure for analysing the qualitative data from the diary-interview schedules, the focused-interview schedules and the substantive and preanalytical field notes was adapted from Burnard (1991).

RESEARCH FINDINGS

A number of themes relating directly to the clinical autonomy of the CPN in the CMHT (and her or his role in general) emerged from the analysis of the quantitative and qualitative data. The measurement of the CPNs' levels of clinical autonomy is centred upon the forms of action that were taken with the 252 new clients received over the 2 years during which data were collected.

The most frequent referral source (see Table 6.1 for percentage breakdowns) was the general practitioner (98 referrals) and next the consultant psychiatrist or another medical practitioner working with the consultant (57 referrals). Forty-one of the clients were referred by other agencies. This included the staff of local authority residential homes, senior nurses from psychiatric hospital wards where the client was an inpatient or relatives and neighbours of the client. Self-referrals accounted for 19 of the clients. However, the CMHT as a whole only referred two clients.

Table 6.1 Source of referrals

Referrer	Frequency	Percent
Consultant psychiatrist	40	15.9
Other psych	17	6.7
General practitioner	98	38.9
Other medical practitioner	2	0.8
Social worker	3	1.2
Psychologist	3	1.2
CPN	16	6.3
CMHT	2	0.8
Health visitor	6	2.4
Manager	5	2.0
Self-referred	19	7.5
Other	41	16.3
Total	252	100.0

Key: other psych, other member of psychiatric medical team

Table 6.2 The client's mental health problem

Value label	Frequency	Percent
Anxiety	49	19.4
Depression	64	25.4
Phobia	7	2.8
Delusions	7	2.8
Delusions and hallucinations	35	13.9
Confusion	2	0.8
Overactivity	8	3.2
Aggression	5	2.0
Self-harm (actual)	4	1.6
Self-harm (implied)	4	1.6
Drug/alcohol addiction	12	4.8
Problems with living	29	11.5
Sexual problems	4	1.6
Eating problems	2	0.8
Other	20	7.9
Total	252	100.0

The CPNs were asked during the diary-interviews to state what they considered to be the major problem with each of the new referrals (Table 6.2). One-quarter were described as suffering from depression and a fifth from anxiety. Delusions and/or hallucinations were seen by the CPN to be the paramount problem in nearly 17% of the cases. Reasons which either explicitly or implicitly were given as 'problems with living' accounted for over 11% (n = 29) of the referrals.

Expectations of the referrer

The CPNs were asked in the diary-interviews if the person referring the client had stated what kind of treatment (or any other action) she or he wanted to be carried out (Table 6.3). Significantly, the referrers did not indicate what they wanted the CPNs to do for two-fifths of the 252 new clients in this study. Although social workers and the CMHT as a whole referred only three and two clients respectively, for none of these were the referrer's expectations specified. No details of what the referrer expected of the CPN were given for 12 of the 19 self-referrals or for three of the six referrals made by health visitors. Nor were they supplied for 17 of the 41 clients referred by agencies in the classification 'other', two of the five made by the CPNs' managers, one of the three made by psychologists and five of the 16 made by other CPNs.

Of the 98 referrals made by general practitioners, nearly half were referred without any mention of expectations.

Table 6.3 Expectations of referrers (adapted from Barratt 1989)

Value label	Frequency	Percent
Assessment	44	17.5
Counselling	13	5.2
Giving medication	18	7.1
Advising	4	1.6
Specialist therapy	18	7.1
Reassurance/support	25	9.9
Monitoring	14	5.6
Evaluating	1	0.4
Unspecified	102	40.5
Other	13	5.2
Total	252	100.0

Interviewer: *The GP wasn't specific about what he wanted you to do?*

CPN: *Never is. Never. I'd reckon nine out of 10 referrals we get are non-directive.*

Unlike the general practitioners, the consultant psychiatrists made their expectations clear in 32 of their 40 referrals.

The data relating to the expectations of the referrers imply that the CPNs make independent decisions about what type of involvement they will have with clients. This does not, however, imply that they are clinically autonomous. CPNs' control over this aspect of the referral process appears mainly to be the result of a lack of clarity by the referrers on what exactly they want from the CPN. Moreover, what seemed to be the implicit and overriding requirement of the CPN was not that a particular form of clinical intervention took place, but that the referrer was relieved of the problem of dealing with the client.

Accepting clients

There is an apparent indiscriminate acceptance of all referrals by the CPNs. That is, all the referrals were accepted as clients in the sense that they were included in the CPNs' caseload numbers (although some were discharged after a relatively short period of time or were categorized as 'inactive'). None of the CPNs gave the reason for accepting a new referral as having been the result of a formal assessment. Formal assessment forms were used in two of the four teams but even when they were used, they were not referred to as a justification for continuing to be involved with the client, for stopping involvement or for re-referring the client to another health-care professional.

From 252 referrals, only on five occasions did the CPNs state that they had accepted the referral because they believed that they had the specialist skills to deal with the issues for which the referrer had indicated the client needed help or the CPNs themselves decided were the client's problem/illness. Seven of the referrals were accepted by the CPNs because they believed that the individual would be 'interesting to work with'. This the CPNs appeared to conclude subsequent to reading the details on the referral from, having had a conversation with the referrer or following their initial contact with the client.

The CPNs reported that they had accepted only three clients as a result of being identified during CMHT discussions as the practitioners with the relevant skills or experience. Sixteen of the referrals were accepted by the CPNs because they had been clients of that particular CPN service at some time in the past. The client being known to the psychiatric services seemed to be taken as a valid reason for making contact and offering treatment. Thirty-five clients were accepted on the basis that they were delegated (by another health-care professional or a manager) to a named CPN. Nearly one-third of the clients referred in this way were from consultant psychiatrists.

The CPNs accepted nearly one-quarter of the 252 referrals on the basis that they were 'appropriate', without further explanation. There were, however, a number of occasions when a referrer's good record of providing appropriate clients encouraged the CPN to accept subsequent referrals. Most significant of all, however, is that almost half of the referrals were contacted by the CPNs (and the vast majority then placed on their caseloads) for reasons that may be described as 'arbitrary'. Thus, for nearly half of the referrals, the CPN's justification for accepting the referred individual as a client was incidental to such criteria as the apparent appropriateness of the referral, whether or not the CPN possessed the relevant skills or whether or not the referral had been delegated to that particular CPN.

Interviewer: *Why did you accept her?*
CPN: *I don't know with this one, really. My turn, I suppose ...*

The chance reasons for a CPN treating a client may suggest that CPNs are inherently generic and that they behave capriciously in determining who takes a particular referral because in effect it does not matter which CPN provides treatment for which client. Conversely, it could be interpreted as a less than well organized and effective approach to matching available resources to the perceived needs of the clients. However, even when the CPN decides that she or he has the specialist skills, knowledge and/or experience to provide treatment for a client, it does not always seem to be the result of some formal appraisal but merely the CPN's own opinion of her or his abilities or again the product of relatively arbitrary processes.

Interviewer: *Why did you accept the referral?*

CPN: *Um [5 s pause], I tend to take ladies with depression and anxiety problems.*

Accepting a referral therefore appears to be dependent on factors other than the objective testing of a client's suitability to enter into the psychiatric system. Furthermore, it became apparent when talking with the CPNs that they had a considerable amount of freedom to influence the size and shape of their caseloads. For example, a number of clients with whom all active involvement by the CPNs had ceased were kept on their caseloads. Most interesting, however, was that the construction of the CPN's caseloads and the creation of psychiatric careers for those individuals referred to the CPNs was influenced by the CPN's decision to either visit or not visit the general practitioners' surgeries.

CPN: *I try to control the amount of referrals, you know, from the GPs, I get by not visiting their surgeries so often.*

The rate of referrals to the CPNs by the general practitioners depends to a significant extent, therefore, on the number of times the surgeries are attended. Furthermore, certain general practitioners are targeted by the CPNs when new referrals are required to increase caseloads, i.e. those who have a track record of supplying what the CPNs perceive as 'appropriate' clients. Alternatively, although referrals could still be delivered by post, CPNs can moderate their physical attendance at general practitioners' surgeries as a method of avoiding direct pressure to take on more clients.

Discussions with colleagues

What became obvious from the early stages of the study was that the CPNs did not appear to talk regularly with colleagues or managers about any aspect of their work with clients. For two-thirds of the 1712 weeks reviewed in the study, the CPNs did not discuss the clients with anyone at all. That is, in less than one-third of the weeks covered in the research did the CPNs communicate directly with, for example, a colleague about the assessment, treatment, prognosis or discharge of the 252 new clients. The CPNs had the most discussions with general practitioners (one-fifth) and then consultant psychiatrists (13%). This was to be expected given that these two groups provided the majority of the referrals.

With respect to indirect communication, the CPNs and their managers stated that it was necessary to supply a new client's general practitioner with a letter indicating what treatment was being offered and another letter when the client was discharged. This procedure also applied to the client's psychiatrist, if one was or had been involved. However, on only 51 occasions did the CPNs report that this had happened.

Where the psychiatrists or general practitioners referred a client, discussions were more likely to occur. However, the clients who had been referred by the consultant psychiatrist were less likely to be discussed by the CPNs than those referred by the general practitioners.

The next most frequent set of discussions were with other CPNs. These were held on 87 (11.4%) occasions. This, however, is a very low figure considering that all but one of the CPNs shared an office with at least one other CPN. That is, it could be assumed that informal discussions about clients would be an inevitable occurrence where CPNs met regularly in the working environment, but the data suggest that this is not the case. Discussions with staff belonging to the psychiatric medical teams (apart from the consultant psychiatrists) were held on 55 occasions (7.2%). Other conferment took place between the CPNs and:

◆ occupational therapists on 43 occasions (5.7%)
◆ social workers on 22 occasions (2.9%)
◆ psychologists on 10 occasions (0.6%)
◆ managers on 12 occasions (1.6%)
◆ supervisors on two occasions (0.3%).

The overall lack of discussion did not seem to concern the CPNs. Indeed, they appeared to deceive themselves about how much contact they actually had with colleagues as they often stated that it was their normal practice to consult constantly with, for example, the consultant psychiatrists, general practitioners or the membership of the CMHT as a whole, before accepting or discharging a client. As the data indicate (from the CPNs' own accounts of what they did with each specific client), this did not happen. Other members of the CMHT were not under any such misapprehension. The psychiatrists in particular complained that the CPNs did not discuss the clients. However, in turn, the CPNs criticized the consultant psychiatrists for not always being accessible.

Discharge and assessment

Nearly one-third (81) of the clients in this study were discharged. A further 29 (11.5%) were re-referred to another professional in the field of mental health and were subjected to a similar process to that involved in the discharge of clients. As we have seen in the section above, the CPNs did not discuss their clients regularly with colleagues. Almost without exception, the CPNs in this study made the decision to discharge, and frequently carried out the discharge, without discussion with any other colleague. Moreover, any discussion that took place happened after the decision to discharge the client had been made. The consultant psychiatrist and general practitioner are told of the CPN's intention to discharge the client or are informed of the discharge after it has occurred.

> Interviewer: *So, you've actually discharged her [the client]?*
> CPN: *Yes, yeah.*
> Interviewer: *Have you done anything after the discharge, have you discussed her with anyone?*
> CPN: *No, no. I'll write a letter to the GP.*

Many of the CPNs' colleagues were very critical of the way in which clients were discharged, as the following quote from one of the consultant psychiatrists illustrates.

> *I'd prefer to be informed before it's done. Ideally I like to get the message, 'I think this person is ready for discharge, and I'd like to discuss it with you', rather than somebody phoning me and saying 'I've discharged Fred Bloggs'.*

Decisions to discharge were taken not only without any discussion with colleagues, but also no formal or objective criteria were reported as being used to evaluate the effects of the treatment or readiness of the client for discharge. As with a significant proportion of the reasons given for accepting clients, decisions to discharge appeared to be subjective and arbitrary.

> Interviewer: *What did you do for that three-quarters of an hour [with the client]?*
> CPN: *We reviewed what we'd done, and what had happened since I'd met him, and if there was any more to be done, and I discharged him.*

The CPNs asserted many times in the diary-interviews that for the first session with a client they would assess her or his mental state and what course of action to take (if any) in the future. Two-thirds of the 44 clients whom the referrers had asked specifically to be assessed by the CPN were seen in the first week following the referral being made. Twenty-three of these 29 were described by the CPNs as having been assessed. However, out of the 71.2% (n = 178) of the clients monitored in the study who were seen in the first week, only three-fifths of these were assessed according to the CPNs' own elaborate versions of what they did during these initial sessions.

More significantly, on only one-fifth of the total number of occasions when direct contact occurred (n = 706) did the CPNs indicate that they had assessed the client. If the CPNs were assessing each client then this figure should have been at the very least the same as the number of clients in the study (i.e. 252) and probably much higher given the CPNs' claims that they may take more than one week to complete the task of assessment.

Discord in the team

In all four teams participating in this research there was considerable confusion about both the functions and status of the CMHT and the roles of its participants. For example, 'leaders' were never expressly identified in any of the teams. In two of the teams, the term 'coordinator' was used to describe the person who accepted the responsibility of arranging and acting as chairperson for meetings, but who held no authority to direct the practice of the other members. With respect to leadership, the opinions of the consultant psychiatrists were unequivocal, as the following quote from one consultant psychiatrist demonstrates.

I think the consultant is the person to actually lead a team, which includes the CPNs ...

As has been found in other studies (Onyett et al 1994), conflict occurs in CMHTs when psychiatrists attempt to dominate other team members. A large part of the discord between the CPNs and consultant psychiatrists, however, relates specifically to the existence of an 'open' referral system. This system, supported by the nursing management, encouraged a high rate of referrals to be sent directly to the CPNs from general practitioners and thereby reduced the psychiatrists' sphere of influence over the work of the CPNs. Consultant psychiatrists felt that such a system created difficulties in identifying who had medical responsibility for the client.

However, the CPNs are in a double bind with respect to medical responsibility and clinical autonomy. On the one hand, nine of the 10 CPNs stated that they wanted to accept whichever clients they find appropriate and from whatever source. But on the other hand, all the CPNs want a psychiatrist or a general practitioner to accept 'medical' responsibility, which appeared to be a euphemism for 'ultimate' liability. That is, in the final analysis, the medical staff would be expected to 'carry the can' for the clients on the CPNs' caseloads.

Resisting dominance

The CPNs do not always passively accept the manoeuvres of psychiatrists to dominate their clinical practice. During the interviews for this research, their response to the consultant psychiatrists stipulating what treatment they expected to be implemented was often one of expressed hostility. In the quotation below, the CPN recalls being asked by the consultant psychiatrist to visit a client who had 'absconded' from hospital after having been admitted following an attempt at suicide. The consultant wanted the CPN to ensure that the client had not injured herself.

I did two visits, neither of which was answered. So, I got back to the consultant and explained the situation, and said 'I've been back twice, how many times would you like me to continue trying to trace this girl?' ... It seemed to me that I was going to have to clear up someone else's inefficiency if you like. She'd been an inpatient in hospital, she'd taken an overdose, why wasn't she observed? Why wasn't she kept an eye on if she was at risk? I was annoyed, because I felt I was being used if you like, and I also felt that it was an inappropriate referral for a CPN anyway. Why didn't they ring the social worker?

As with the issue of medical responsibility, a double bind of the CPN's own making exists with respect to occupational status. That is, whilst complaining about being used by the consultant psychiatrist to 'clear up someone else's inefficiency', the CPN does not refuse the request. Whatever the moral argument for visiting the client in these circumstances, doing so has the effect of reinforcing the CPN's subservient role to the consultant psychiatrist. Moreover, the introduction of 'supervision registers' (NHS Management Executive 1994) and the enforced return into hospital care of some mentally ill people under the 1995 Mental Health (Patients in the Community) Act underline the capacity of the psychiatrist to dictate significant elements of the CPN's role.

Supervision

Although in this study there was little clarity about what sort of supervision should be adopted (i.e. 'managerial' supervision or 'developmental' supervision), most of the CPNs, their colleagues and the managers regarded supervision to be of importance. Key questions included the type of supervision CPNs undertook and whether it was available on an informal or formal basis. The terms 'formal' and 'informal' are used to differentiate between regular pre-organized (and normally obligatory) sessions with an identified supervisor and *ad hoc* discussions with any available colleague (Box 6.2).

In the early part of the study, six of the 10 CPNs stated that they received formal supervision from one of their colleagues in the CMHT or from a manager. All 10 of the CPNs in the study stated that they undertook frequent

---

Box 6.2 Defining Supervision

The supervision of health-care practitioners has become a major concern internationally (Severinsson 1995). In the United Kingdom, there is much discussion about how to incorporate supervision into nursing practice (Jones 1996, Morcom & Hughes 1996). There are, however, numerous definitions of supervision (Hawkings & Shohet 1989, Wilkin cited in Butterworth & Faugier 1992, Department of Health 1994). Two of the most obvious are, first, the form of interaction which is connected with managerial control and second, the type which is associated with the reviewing of clinical work in order to help the personal development and/or the skills of the practitioner being supervised.

informal supervision on demand, usually from another CPN (especially if sharing an office with that CPN), but occasionally from a colleague who belonged to one of the other occupational groups. However, contradicting the initial impression given by the CPNs, the data from the whole of the study indicate that formal supervision (managerial or developmental) was provided on only two occasions.

Furthermore, later in the study, the CPNs admitted that although supervision officially was expected to take place, it generally did not. Observations conducted during the study showed that the CPNs do talk with other nursing colleagues in the team about their clients in a general way on many occasions. But mostly the clients are mentioned in conversations which cover other non-related topics. For example, a client's treatment or prognosis may be alluded to in the middle of a discussion about the CPNs' working conditions or personal circumstances. Therefore, it would be difficult to classify these communications as even 'informal' supervision.

Role of CPNs

A lot of people are asking at the moment 'What is the role of the CPN?'. I think a lot of people are starting to say 'These are expensive people, what are they doing?'. (Manager)

The role of the CPN, as described by the CPNs, their colleagues in the CMHT and their managers, is not well defined. That is, the informants in the study were unable to provide a lucid definition of the part played by the CPN in mental health care. However, one common theme reported by the CPNs' colleagues was that they considered a constituent of the CPN role was administering and monitoring medication and in particular the giving of major tranquillizers by injection to people suffering from long-term mental illness.

The CPNs were somewhat ambivalent about this aspect of their work. When they believed it to be justified (for example, if the condition of a client was considered to be in danger of deteriorating without medication), this task would be performed unquestioningly. However, at other times they complained that they did not wish to be 'used' by the medical practitioners for this purpose. They argued that the administering of injections could be carried out by, for example, district nurses or nurses employed by general practitioners. The CPNs seemed to regard the giving of injections to the mentally ill as a waste of their expertise – an 'expertise' they consistently failed to define.

It has been argued for some time that CPNs are abandoning altogether their attachment to working with the chronically mentally ill (Weleminsky 1989, personal communication). Much criticism was levelled at the CPNs in this study by psychiatrists about neglecting this group of clients, particularly those suffering from schizophrenia. It was suggested that the CPNs had become too embroiled with the client group described as the 'worried well'. The clients in this group are principally those who have been diagnosed as suffering from neurotic illnesses and who are mainly referred directly to the CPNs by the general practitioners. A specific criticism from one psychiatrist was that the CPNs (and 'other' practitioners in the team) want to work only with 'interesting' and 'rewarding' clients and not those who suffer from psychotic illness.

> It's great for CPNs to do, or other professionals to do, support groups for unmarried mothers and things which is fine, but here we've got a high percentage of chronic, severely mentally ill people and in my book they come first. The well people who are worried are in need of help but the chronically mentally ill have to come first because they're the most vulnerable basically ... what can happen is that all the exciting and interesting and rewarding things get done and the chronics get left to fester basically.

This concern about the CPNs concentrating too much on primary prevention and referrals from general practitioners was echoed by one of the nurse managers. This manager described working with the chronically mentally ill as the 'bread and butter' of psychiatric nursing, an area of work that shouldn't be left behind because CPNs have got the 'skills that nobody else has got'.

The role of the CPN, therefore, whilst lacking in clarity, is perceived to encompass a number of exclusive facets. The CPN is identified by her or his colleagues with the giving and supervising of medication. Although the CPN is viewed as having steered away from treating the chronically mentally disturbed, this is considered still to be an area of work that the CPN should tackle.

DISCUSSION

With respect to clinical autonomy, the CPNs in this study exercised a high degree of independence in their working practices. However, ability to work unhindered does not necessarily indicate the existence of genuine autonomy. That is, the CPNs have not achieved their clinical autonomy through a successful campaign of occupational advancement aimed at achieving the status of 'professionals'. They have autonomy because what they do in their practice has been left unobserved and unmanaged. One of the managers interviewed in the study, apparently unaware of her own responsibilities for overseeing the work of her subordinates, was candid about how isolated the CPNs are.

> CPNs make decisions about clinical situations that they have to deal with, often without consultation with anyone else, not necessarily by design but often because there isn't anybody else to consult with.

Managerial negligence

The limited management control over the work of the CPNs has considerable impact on the delivery of the psychiatric services. For example, although the CPNs do not prevent an individual referred to them from becoming a 'client' of the psychiatric system (because they accept all referrals onto their caseloads), they do adjudicate over who should and should not be labelled 'mentally ill'. They do this when they decide whether to attend general practitioners' surgeries. That is, a patient of a general practitioner could become a client of the psychiatric services as a result of a CPN realizing that she or he is in need of a larger caseload.

Moreover, the way in which they work has a major influence on the 'psychiatric careers' of their clients. CPNs in this study regulated the length of time clients remained within the psychiatric system and the type of treatment offered on the basis of capricious and unsupervised decisions. In particular, CPNs appear to discharge clients not only without any prior discussion with colleagues, supervisors or managers but also without reference to any objective evaluation of the clients' fitness for discharge.

Potential for disaster

This latter practice has been condemned in the Ritchie Report (1994), which examined the circumstances that led to the murder of Jonathan Zito by Christopher Clunis. Clunis (diagnosed as a paranoid schizophrenic) killed Jonathan Zito on a London Underground platform in December 1992. The attention of the media has also been drawn to criticism of 'unrefined' practices by mental health workers.

> *The body of a mentally ill man was found in his council flat weeks after he died and nearly six months after he was last seen by his community psychiatric nurse an inquest heard ... Malcolm McDuff ... had not had his monthly injection to control his schizophrenia since last December. Police found his body lying in an armchair last week, after being called in by neighbours who had not seen Mr McDuff for over a month.* (Brindle 1994)

This is not to suggest that any of the 10 CPNs in the study were involved in serious professional misjudgements. Furthermore, inquiries and media reports into homicides by the mentally ill highlight the failings of practitioners other than nurses. However, lax practices by psychiatric nurses have the potential to lead to disaster when and if the 'right' circumstances transpire (Box 6.3).

Rigour in practice

What, then, can be recommended to improve CPN practice? David Skidmore (1984) described CPNs as being skilled practitioners of the 'art of muddling

> **Box 6.3** The reality of schizophrenic homicide rates
>
> It is worth noting that only a small number of people labelled mentally ill are aggressive either to others or to themselves. People diagnosed schizophrenic are much more likely to commit suicide than homicide (Boyd 1996). The number of homicides carried out by 'normal' people is growing, whereas the homicide rate amongst the mentally ill is relatively static or even in decline (Muijen 1997).

through'. Although many educational initiatives have been put in place since Skidmore called for CPNs to be given extensive training '… in the interest of both client and nurse' (Skidmore 1984), it would seem that a sharp definition of their function remains elusive.

CPNs may be described as the 'artful dodgers' of the mental health world. They have expanded only by stealing roles previously belonging to other occupations without quite knowing what to do when they have them. (Sheppard 1991)

In order to ensure rigour in the practice of community psychiatric nursing, there are a number of recommendations for the role of the CPN in the CMHT (adapted from Morral 1997b).

Discharge

The 1995 Mental Health (Patients in the Community) Act legislates for 'compulsory supervision' of certain inpatients on discharge from hospital into the community. CPNs, where they are the key workers, will have to implement formalized care plans. This should prevent the arbitrary removal of these service users from the CPN's caseload. It is suggested by the Department of Health (1996) that care plans should be reviewed by all of those involved with their delivery. The author suggests that no client should be discharged from the CPN's caseload or re-referred to another agency or professional unless this is first discussed by the CMHT and agreed upon by the leader of the team. As recommended by Blom-Cooper et al (1995), 'essential documentation', in the form of a written evaluation of the client's mental state and social circumstances, should be produced before the client is discharged or re-referred. The notion of a 'discharge contract', made between the CPN and the service user, could be considered (House of Commons Health Committee 1994).

Supervision

Supervision has been identified as essential to the work of mental health nurses (Department of Health 1994). The responsibility for the supervision of the clinical work of the mental health nurse working in the community should be taken over by the leader of the CMHT. The team leader could appoint another 'senior' practitioner to conduct the supervision, but should retain overall responsibility for ensuring that an effective process is put into operation. To be effective, supervision should be mandatory (i.e. enshrined in the CPN's contract with their employing health authority or NHS trust), as well as being both 'managerial' and 'developmental'.

Authority and responsibility

The CMHTs in this study could be viewed as operating merely as a loose network of mental health practitioners, rather than as a cohesive 'team'. As Boyd (1996) suggests, teams require unambiguous lines of accountability and authority.

The author agrees with the report into mental health nursing, Working in Partnership (Department of Health 1994), that protocols defining the roles and responsibilities of each member, discipline or agency should be produced. Moreover, as is suggested in the Sainsbury Centre's review of the training of mental health practitioners (Sainsbury Centre 1997), core competencies across specialisms must be identified. In particular, the role of the CPN '... should be more clearly defined' (Audit Commission 1994).

CONCLUSION

The nurses in the study appear to organize their caseloads in a way that can be characterized as arbitrary. That is, the CPNs do not ordinarily assess the needs of the clients effectively and in the main do not receive (or do not accept) guidance from the referrers about what form of treatment may be appropriate. Furthermore, the CPNs would appear to discharge clients without any objective evaluation of how ready they are for this action to be taken. This is a particularly pertinent finding given the current lay opinion climate, which questions the positive impact of community care or at least the placement of clients with diagnoses such as schizophrenia or personality disorder in community settings.

The CPNs also adopt specific techniques to manipulate the size of their caseloads and do not discuss their clients on a regular basis with the person who made the referral in the first instance, managers or with their colleagues in the CMHT. This is the case even when the CPN has decided to discharge a client. Formal or informal supervision does not appear to exist on a regular basis.

Relationships between the CPNs and their colleagues in the CMHT are reported to be characterized at times by interdisciplinary hostility. This is focused in particular upon the consultant psychiatrists' attempts to attain or retain dominance. But the CPNs do use covert techniques to avoid their work being directed by psychiatrists. The potential for psychiatrists to dominate CPNs was undermined further by the latter accepting referrals from general practitioners and self-referrals.

Opinions vary amongst the members of the CMHT and the managers about the role of the CPN. However, there does seem to be common agreement about one specific element – the giving and monitoring of medication.

In a rapidly changing and unpredictable world, the role of the CPN will not remain static. It will constantly adjust and evolve. However, whatever the professional aspirations of the discipline are and no matter how much society vacillates in its demands on mental health nurses, there must be safeguards to protect a vulnerable group like the mentally ill from deleterious practices.

The work of community psychiatric nurses must be open to scrutiny. It is crucial, however, that nurses working in the community do not come under the observation of their colleagues or managers to anything like the extent they do when they work inside hospitals. Moreover, the formal auditing of clinical work cannot easily compensate for the inherently 'concealed' work of community staff. Consequently, more sophisticated mechanisms must be developed to achieve national standards for sustaining competent performance (Sainsbury Centre 1997). These mechanisms must also be capable of evaluating whether or not standards are being met and guarantee that corrective action is taken if this is not the case.

QUESTIONS FOR DISCUSSION

◆ How much autonomy should CPNs have to carry out their work?

◆ What procedures can be used to ensure that the needs of psychiatric service users are being met by CPNs?

◆ What might be the 'core competencies' of the CPN?

ANNOTATED BIBLIOGRAPHY

Morrall P A 1998 Mental health nursing and social control. Whurr, London

This text outlines the research study described above which is explored in more detail. It includes a comprehensive review of the literature relating to the status of nursing in general and psychiatric nursing in particular. The role of the mental health nurse in the 'social control' of the 'mad' is also evaluated. The text argues for (some) mental health nurses to become part of a radical force aimed at achieving genuine empowerment for the mentally disordered.

Ovretviet J 1993 Coordinating community care: multidisciplinary teams and care management. Open University Press, Buckingham.

Ovretveit gives practical advice on how to work more effectively in community teams. For example, he tackles the problem of bringing together a range of disciplines and agencies, each of which may have its own methods of work and philosophy. The author's aim is to help make the most of the different skills the various practitioners bring to a multidisciplinary team in order to 'make community care a reality'.

Rogers A, Pilgrim D, Lacey R 1993 Experiencing psychiatry: users' views of services. Macmillan/Mind, London

This book recounts users' experiences of the mental health services. It provides an invaluable insight into what people suffering from mental illness think of hospitals, community provision and the treatments (for example, electroconvulsant therapy and major tranquillizers) they receive.

REFERENCES

Armstrong J 1987 Community health nurses – the frontline workers. Canadian Journal of Psychiatric Nursing 28 (4): 4–6

Audit Commission 1994 Finding a place: a review of mental health services for adults. HMSO, London

Barratt E 1989 Community psychiatric nurses: their self-perceived roles. Journal of Advanced Nursing 14: 42–48

Blom-Cooper L, Hally H, Murphy E 1995 The falling shadow: one patient's mental health care 1978–1993. Duckworth, London

Boyd W 1996 (chairperson) Report of the confidential inquiry into homicides and suicides by mentally ill people. Royal College of Psychiatrists, London

Brindle D 1994 Schizophrenic's death fuels community care fear. The Guardian, 2 June

Burgess R G 1981 Keeping a research diary. Cambridge Journal of Education 11 (1): 75–83

Burnard P 1991 A method of analysing interview scripts in qualitative research. Nurse Education Today 11: 461–466

Butterworth T, Faugier J (eds) 1992 Clinical supervision and mentorship in nursing. Chapman & Hall, London

Department of Health 1994 Working in partnership: a collaborative approach to care. Report of the mental health nursing review team (chairperson T Butterworth). HMSO, London

Department of Health 1996 The spectrum of care: local services for people with mental health problems. Department of Health, London

Ezard J 1997 Internet creating computer junkies. The Guardian, 7 August

Fletcher D 1995 Care of mentally ill in state of turmoil. Electronic Telegraph, 25 August

Freidson E 1970 Professional dominance: the social structure of medical care. Aldine, Chicago

Freidson E 1988 The profession of medicine: a study of the sociology of applied knowledge – with a new afterword. University of Chicago Press, Chicago

Hally H 1989 All in a day's work. Community outlook 6–11 January: 4–6

Hawkings P, Shohet R 1989 Supervision in the helping professions. Open University Press, Buckingham

House of Commons Health Committee 1994 Better off in the community? The care of people who are seriously mentally ill, Vol 1. HMSO, London

Jones A 1996 Clinical supervision: a framework for practice. International Journal of psychiatric nursing research 3 (1): 290–307

Jones S G (ed) 1995 Cybersociety: computer-mediated communication and community. Sage, London

Mihill C 1997 Computers 'cause social conversation to come unstuck'. The Guardian, 16 July

Morcom C, Hughes R 1996 How can clinical supervision become a real vision for the future? Journal of Psychiatric and Mental Health Nursing 3: 117–124

Morrall P A 1997a Interpersonal communication in cybersociety. Paper presented to the Australian and New Zealand College of Mental Health Nurses Conference, Communication in Practice, Adelaide, Australia.

Morrall P A 1997b Lacking in rigour: a case-study of the professional practice of psychiatric nurses in four community mental health teams. Journal of Mental Health 6 (2): 173–179

Morrall P A 1998 Mental health nursing and social control. Whurr, London

Muijen M 1997 A man for all reasons. The Guardian (Society), 8 October

NHS Management Executive 1994 Introduction of supervision registers for mentally ill people from April 1994. HMSO, London

Onyett S, Heppleston T, Bushnell D 1994 A national survey of community mental health teams. Team structures and process. Journal of Mental Health 3: 175–194

Peplau H E 1994 Psychiatric mental health nursing: challenge and change. Journal of Psychiatric and Mental Health Nursing 1 (1): 3–7

Ritchie J H 1994 (chairperson) The report of the inquiry into the care and treatment of Christopher Clunis. Presented to the Chairman of North East Thames and South East Thames Regional Health Authorities. HMSO, London

Sainsbury Centre 1997 Pulling together: the future roles and training of mental health staff. Sainsbury Centre for Mental Health, London

Severinsson E I 1995 Clinical supervision in health care. Nordic School of Public Health, Goteborg, Sweden

Sheppard M 1991 Mental health work in the community. Falmer Press, London

Skidmore D 1984 Community psychiatric nursing: muddling through. Nursing times (community outlook) May 9: 179–181

7

The emergence and development of practice nursing – implications for future policy and practice

Neil Lunt   Karl Atkin

KEY ISSUES

◆ The emergence of practice nurses as a new professional group.

◆ Role and management: marrying professionalism with a diverse clinical portfolio.

◆ Training and education: preventing fragmentation and moving away from task-based development.

◆ Future development and the centrality of practice nursing to primary health-care provision.

INTRODUCTION

This chapter explores the emergence and development of practice nurses as a professional group. *It traces the emergence of practice nurses and discusses their role, training and future development. It specifically explores five policy questions:

◆ Why, given the unplanned growth of practice nursing, did GPs choose to employ practice nurses?

---

* The work is based on a wider study commissioned by the Department of Health and Welsh Office to inform their strategy on practice nursing (Atkin et al 1993, Atkin & Lunt 1996a,b)

◆ What expectations do GPs have of the practice nurse role?
◆ What role do practice nurses undertake and what training issues does this raise?
◆ What are the nurses' and GPs' future aspirations for the development of practice nursing?
◆ How do health commissioners and community nurse managers view the emergence of practice nursing and what implications does this have for health policy developments?

Ten years ago, nurses employed in general practice under the direction of general practitioners were comparatively rare. Changes in UK health policy and in the delivery of community health services, however, have led to a growth in their numbers. Since 1988, the number of whole-time equivalents (WTEs) has trebled and most practices now employ at least one practice nurse (Atkin et al 1993). There are in the region of 15 000 practice nurse posts in England and Wales, representing around 9400 whole-time equivalents (Hirst et al 1994). In comparison there are 12˜600 health visitor WTEs and 19 090 district nurse WTEs. Therefore, practice nurses – although fewer in number than district nurses and health visitors – represent a substantial primary health-care resource.

By the early 1990s there was little research-based evidence available, on a national level, that explored the practice nurse role. This was despite the substantial growth in practice nurse numbers and the large amount of health funding spent on this growth. Estimates from 1994, for example, suggest that it cost a typical FHSA with almost 100 WTE practice nurses, around two million pounds a year (Atkin & Hirst 1994). Although we do not want to enter intricate and controversial health economic debates, we present such figures merely to emphasize that practice nursing accounts for a substantial proportion of the primary health-care budget. This in itself justifies interest in their emergence and development. To this extent, it is no longer possible to regard practice nursing as an issue of marginal concern to health-care policy.

The rapid growth in practice nurse numbers and the increasing policy emphasis on primary health care raise a series of pressing policy questions around their role, professional preparation and future development (Atkin & Lunt 1996a). This debate necessarily needs to reflect the accounts of different 'stakeholders' with an interest in practice nursing (see Chapter 1). These stakeholders include the nurses themselves and their employing GPs, along with those who have responsibility for managing and purchasing community health services. Evaluating these different accounts within a policy and empirical context are fundamental to understanding the emergence and development of practice nursing.

EVALUATING THE EMERGENCE AND DEVELOPMENT OF PRACTICE NURSING

The evaluation offered by this chapter does not give a simple description of practice nursing, cataloguing the experiences of the main stakeholders, but attempts to locate debates about practice nursing within current policy and practice contexts. Such an approach is seen as especially valuable in informing thinking and practice (Levick 1992). Following this, there are two interrelated aspects informing the evaluative discussion adopted in this chapter. The first involves understanding the policy and practice context informing the emergence and development of practice nursing. Among other things, this understanding explains the importance of exploring the accounts of different stakeholders. The second is concerned with providing an evaluative methodology able to use these policy and practice changes as a basis for informing empirical research.

THE POLICY CONTEXT

The rapid growth in the number of practice nurses has a particular historical context. The growth of practice nurses cannot be understood without examining that context and the changing place of general practice. Amendments to the general practitioner contract in 1966 established the potential for employing practice nurses and some GPs took advantage of this by employing nursing staff to undertake 'treatment room' tasks (Reedy et al 1976). Nonetheless, by the early 1980s, directly employed nurses in general practice remained rare, numbering fewer than 2000 WTEs (Stilwell 1988). Three general policy shifts explain their growth.

First, amendments to the GP system of payments and associated incentives in 1990 created an expanded role for nurses in general practice (Robinson et al 1993). The contract placed new responsibilities on general practitioners. Much of the work specified in the new contract – immunizations, cervical cytology, child surveillance, health promotion, chronic disease management, new registration checks and health assessments of people over 75 – could be performed by appropriately trained nurses (Damant et al 1994). In the period prior to the introduction of the revised contract and immediately afterwards there was a significant growth in the number of nurses directly employed in general practice.

Second, there were particular financial circumstances that encouraged this growth. GPs were particularly attracted to the idea of directly employing a nurse to meet their contractual obligations (Robinson et al 1993). At the same time, reimbursement of practice staff costs by FHSAs followed nationally set regulations in accordance with a non-cash limited budget (Statutory

Instruments 1990). With encouragement from the FHSA, GPs were able to obtain funding for a practice nurse salary with few or no financial restrictions (Atkin & Hirst 1994). Central government implicitly sanctioned this arrangement by choosing not to intervene in the process until 1992 when they introduced cash-limited budgets on the reimbursement of practice staff. By this time, most practices employed at least one practice nurse. The financial framework for expanding the number of practice nurses thus existed and in association with the policy developments described above, stimulated the growth of practice nurse numbers (Atkin & Lunt 1996b). Consequently, practice nursing grew largely in response to the needs of general practice and the provision of general medical services (Ross et al 1994). As such, practice nurses are neither commissioned nor provided in the same way as other primary health-care services.

Third, and more generally, the conditions enabling the growth of practice nursing were not accidental (see also Chapter 1). Government policy has sought to shift the focus of provision from secondary to primary health care and general practice was ideally placed as the organizational base from which to provide these services (Atkin & Lunt 1996a). Large acute hospitals were seen as beset by spiralling financial costs and inappropriate bureaucratic, centralized hierarchies, as well as being insensitive to the needs of the patient (Hoggett 1991). General practice offered a possible solution to these problems by providing flexibility, greater efficiency and 'customer'-orientated health care (NHS Management Executive 1993). The employment of practice nurses was seen to increase this flexibility, thus emphasizing their importance to the successful development of primary health care.

The role of practice nursing

The organizational and policy developments outlined above provide the general context in which more specific debates about practice nursing occur. Beyond this, however, there are a series of specific policy questions about the role of practice nursing in primary health care. This debate touches on a series of interrelated themes including the appropriate role model for practice nurses to adopt and their relationship to other community nurses. How should practice nursing be funded? How should practice nurses be managed? How should their education and training needs be met?

Amendments to the GP contract only provided a general framework, within which practice nursing developed. Consequently, there are considerable variations in the roles performed by practice nurses (Hirst et al 1994). The literature suggests that practice nurses work to a range of role models. Some work within a traditional model of a treatment room nurse; others are developing additional aspects to their work such as chronic disease management or home visits; others see themselves as nurse practitioners providing specialist nursing requiring independent judgement and action (Atkin et al 1993, Audit Commission 1993, Robinson et al 1993).

Whatever role a practice nurse adopts, it is possible that some areas of his/her practice will overlap with the responsibilities of other community-based nurses. Fluid boundaries, although traditionally characterizing community nursing (Robinson 1990), do create the potential for role overlap and duplication, as well as tensions between different types of nurses (Ross 1991). This potential for role overlap raises more general issues about grade and skill mix in primary health care. A more systematic approach to establishment setting is offered as a solution to the difficulties of securing complementary nursing services (Lightfoot et al 1992). Practice nurses, however, have different employers from other community nurses and this arrangement represents different lines of accountability and different philosophies of practice. The expanding role of practice nursing in primary health care and its relationship to other forms of community nursing also raise more obvious questions about teamworking (Poulton & West 1993a,b).

Cost-effectiveness has been given increasing prominence in the current changes, raising questions about the appropriate use of resources in primary health care (Audit Commission 1993). The growth of practice nursing, as we have seen, was not directly managed by central government. Consequently, there are variations in the distribution of the practice nurse resource and allocation is not necessarily related to patient need (Hirst et al 1998). Health-care agencies responsible for reimbursing part of the nurses' salary are considering a more equitable distribution of resources in primary health care (Atkin & Lunt 1996a).

The principal employer of most practice nurses is the general practitioner. However, district health authorities, since their merger with FHSAs, usually reimburse a large proportion of a practice nurse's salary. This arrangement raises questions about how practice nurses should be managed (Martin 1992). At present GPs manage practice nurses; the arrangement, however, is far from clearcut, as health commissioners can assume a more managerial role. Many organizations, for example, have workers to cater for the growing numbers of practice nurses and to plan their role in primary health care. Some authorities, for instance, have refused reimbursement unless a practice nurse is given a job description or a specified number of study days. Health commissioners can also have a say in the quality of work undertaken by practice nurses, for example, by agreeing guidelines for the delivery of care within a practice.

Finally, there is no recognized practice nurse qualification. Most nurses are trained to RGN level. Their postbasic training, however, is somewhat *ad hoc* (Atkin & Lunt 1996b) and this has led many writers to call for a coherent education and training strategy for practice nursing (NHS Management Executive

1993). Appropriate training and education should ensure that practice nurses are properly qualified and trained for the tasks they undertake (Selby et al 1992). Training and education can also enable practice nurses to develop their role (Atkin et al 1993).

The different stakeholders

The policy context which informs the emergence and development of practice nursing generates various stakeholders. Understanding the accounts of these different stakeholders is fundamental in providing an evaluation of practice nursing. Primarily, these stakeholders include the practice nurses themselves, the GPs who employ them and those in the DHA who reimburse a large proportion of a practice nurse's salary, provide professional support for primary health-care staff and facilitate the development of primary health-care services. At a broad level there are two further stakeholders often ignored in the discussions about practice nursing – the commissioner or purchaser of primary health care and the provider who is responsible for managing the community nursing service. The policies and practices of these two stakeholders can assume considerable significance for the development and organization of the primary health-care nursing resource. Commissioning authorities, although not responsible for commissioning practice nursing, have to plan for and assess the health-care needs of a given locality. The merger between the FHSA and DHAs gives them a specific interest in practice nursing. Community nursing providers, although without direct managerial control over practice nurses, develop community nursing services within the context of a substantial practice nurse resource. The different interests and perspectives of these various stakeholders, as well as central and local policy directives, determine the nature and character of care offered by practice nurses.

THE EMPIRICAL STUDY

The research project explored the role of practice nursing in primary health care. The first part, completed in February 1993, was a census of practice nurses (Atkin et al 1993). This chapter draws on material generated from the second stage of the project, which complemented the census data by providing a more detailed understanding of the role of the practice nurse as seen by the nurses themselves, by the GPs who employ them and by those responsible for managing, delivering and planning community nursing services. This part of the project was completed in 1995.

The project conducted fieldwork in 10 family health service authority areas (FHSAs) in England and Wales and adopted a qualitative methodology that focused on indepth one-to-one interviews. These interviews were conducted in three types of practice in each of the 10 fieldwork areas: fundholding,

Box 7.1 Types of practice included in the study

30 practices in the study:
  11 fundholding
  19 non-fundholding[1]
  13 practice nurses were employed in single-handed practices[2]
  25 practice nurses were employed in fundholding practices[2]
  19 were employed in non-fundholding practices

[1]One fundholding practice was single handed but part of a fundholding consortium. This did not alter the ratio of single-handed practices to group practices: 10 single-handed practices and 30 group practices.
[2]One nurse worked in a fundholding single-handed practice.

non-fundholding and single handed. Box 7.1 provides details about the types of practices included in the study.

In every practice, all practice nurses and at least one GP were interviewed. To place this material in context, further interviews were undertaken with FHSA managers, a person responsible for providing community nursing and a person responsible for commissioning community nursing. The final sample is listed in Box 7.2.

QUALITATIVE EVALUATION

The practical aspects of the project have been described above. We now provide a more philosophical account which justifies the empirical evaluation adopted by the project.

Evaluation has long been dominated by the conventional or classic approach (see Chapter 1). The principal features are definition of the intervention to be assessed; definable inputs, an experimental and a control group; and measurement of the difference between pre- and postinterventions

Box 7.2 The sample

56 practice nurses
29 general practitioners
11 managers of community provider units
12 commissioners of community nursing
17 FHSA representatives
12 Regional health authority managers
1 Welsh Office representative

(Goldberg & Connelly 1982). Although having an important role to play in research design, conventional approaches to evaluation have been criticized for failing to account for process and different interpretations of social reality (Gubrium & Silverman 1989). This has led to an interest in more 'constructivist' approaches to evaluation (Guba & Lincoln 1989). The aim of 'constructivist' or 'pluralist' evaluation is understanding or *verstehen*, rather than causal inference (Outhwaite 1975). Such an approach denies a single simple social reality, regarding such realities as plural (Smith & Cantley 1985). As such, context is regarded as central to understanding (Mishler 1986).

The pluralist approach to evaluation has been a powerful influence on the approach adopted in this project (Smith & Cantley 1985, Twigg & Atkin 1994). There are two features of pluralist evaluation of particular relevance to this chapter. First, pluralist evaluation recognizes that different stakeholders present different accounts of social reality and that these different accounts do not have the same possibility of being realized. As we have seen, there are various stakeholders with an interest in practice nursing. Each stakeholder attempts to produce a legitimate version of the world and have this recognized by others (Bourdieu 1984). Facts do not speak for themselves but are subject to various interpretations (Guba & Lincoln 1989). Pluralist research enables researchers to understand these different accounts of social reality and explore their influence on policy and practice (Gubrium & Silverman 1989).

Second, pluralist research emphasizes the importance of understanding process rather than simple outcomes (Twigg & Atkin 1994). For example, the work carried out by practice nurses included in this study did not differ from that described in other studies. Much of the earlier research, however, is quantitative and usually asks the respondent to indicate, from a list of predetermined tasks, the type of work she or he is performing (Audit Commission 1993). This approach, although invaluable in representing the work of practice nurses, has been criticized for emphasizing the task-orientated nature of practice nursing rather than the scope of the nurses' work.

Pluralist research helps counter this by enabling researchers to explore the meaning implicit in the responses of the main stakeholders. This approach, for instance, can provide a more detailed understanding of how the practice nurse's work is organized and the various influences that determine his/her role (Atkin & Lunt 1996a).

The approach to evaluation adopted by this project required a methodology that could reflect the plurality of social reality and accept that different stakeholders utilize and adopt different views in their attempt to make sense of the world. To accommodate this, the empirical component of the evaluation is qualitative, because such a method can provide a basis for understanding complex behaviours and interactions in a way quantitative techniques cannot

(Mishler 1986). The particular strength of qualitative research lies in its ability to allow understanding of process and meaning within a contextual framework and thus enable particular contingent situations to be explained (Gubrium & Silverman 1989). There are various approaches to qualitative methods including focus groups, indepth interviews, observation techniques and document analysis. One-to-one interviews were felt to be the most important way of collecting the information, rather than focus groups. We wanted to understand the workings of each general practice 'unit' and the roles of each of the participants within that unit.

There are different types of interview approach we could have pursued: structured questions that elicit open-ended responses; semistructured that pursue particular themes in an open way; oral history and ethnographic approaches (Hammersley & Atkinson 1983). For the demands of policy research, the approach adopted was to make the interviews semistructured, the style of which could be described as a focused conversation (Merton & Kendal 1946). A topic guide identified a number of key subject areas around which to form questions during the interview. Under each topic, particular probes were included to make the conversation more precise, detailed and concrete. The interviews lasted, on average, 45 min. The interviewer transcribed the tapes into a detailed resumé according to analytical headings. Analysis of these resumés enabled the researcher to define concepts, seek patterns, understand ranges, find linkages and give explanations.

THE RESEARCH FINDINGS

The emergence of practice nursing

The emergence of practice nursing is central to understanding their current role and future development. Drawing on the GPs' accounts, it is possible to identify four demand factors for employing a practice nurse: dissatisfaction with community nursing services; delegation of workload; practice development; and being able to define the work of a nurse.

Dissatisfaction with community nursing services, especially district nursing services, was a key factor in directly employing nursing staff. Many GPs felt community nurses would have difficulty in helping the practice meet the targets specified in the 1990 GP contract. It is, however, important to be clear about the precise focus of GPs' criticisms. They had few problems with the quality of the community nursing services, but instead criticized the range and continuity of provision.

The potential for delegation represented the second reason GPs decided to employ a practice nurse. One single-handed GP, for example, remarked:

Practice nurses must have given us more time ... GPs are far busier than

5 years ago and I don't know how we would have managed without practice nurses.

Most GPs felt practice nurses were able to help with the practice's workload, releasing GP time and improving the general quality of the service offered by the practice.

Third, and closely related to delegation, employment of a practice nurse could help develop the services offered by the practice. Several GPs, for example, had an interest in health promotion but could not follow it up due to lack of surgery time. Practice nurses, however, could provide this service.

Fourth, directly employing a nurse gave GPs the opportunity to define a nurse's role. GPs are able, for example, to delegate tasks to 'their' practice nurse without having to negotiate with community nursing managers. Practice nurses are under their direct control, whereas the community nursing service is not. GPs can therefore decide what work is appropriately performed by themselves and what work is appropriately performed by nurses. Delegation of tasks and a nurse's role in practice development also gives the GP more discretion over how they use their own time in the practice.

More generally, GPs described a range of skills and experience they hoped a practice nurse would have. These include general nursing skills, previous practice nurse experience, the ability to work autonomously and 'personality'. The latter was regarded as especially important. Even when GPs expressed the need for particular skills, these usually included a range of generic skills rather than specific abilities. Similarly, most GPs did not always consider it essential that a nurse was able to perform a particular task, even when the nurse was recruited to do that task. What was more important, from the GPs' point of view, was the nurse's willingness to obtain the necessary training. One GP remarked:

> *Their background doesn't matter as the practice will train them. What is most important is the rapport they have with patients.*

GPs wanted to appoint a nurse who posed no threat to the existing organization of the practice and who could develop and adapt to different roles. Specific skills were less important as they could be acquired; the ability to 'fit in', however, could not.

Becoming a practice nurse

Once the potential of practice nursing had been established, nurses found it an attractive job option. This was evident in their initial reasons for entering practice nursing. These included: dissatisfaction with previous nursing employment; the ability to combine family obligations with nursing employment; and the career opportunities offered by practice nursing. First, and by far the largest group, were those nurses dissatisfied with their previous nursing employment; two-thirds of nurses identified this as instrumental in becoming a practice nurse. The increase in practice nurse posts and the lack of emphasis on formal qualifications provided an alternative form of nursing occupation easily accessible to the respondents. For many of the nurses interviewed, the prime motivation in becoming a practice nurse was connected more with the negative experience of a previous work setting rather than with the definite attractions of practice nursing per se. Hospital nursing, for example, was seen to undermine the exercise of their professional autonomy. Nurses who had previously worked in hospital settings, for example, talked about their 'disillusionment' with working on hospital wards, often feeling deskilled and unable to work on their own initiative. One nurse remarked:

I had no independence on the ward. You could never make decisions on your own. I mean you never knew who your boss was. You had to go through seven line managers to find them.

Second, 12 nurses had been attracted to practice nursing following a break to have children. Practice nursing was perceived as less demanding than hospital nursing and able to offer more flexible working hours. It enabled them to combine nursing employment with caring for a family in a way that a hospital or community setting could not. Several practice nurses with young families, for example, pointed to the attractions of not having to work shifts and weekends. Finally, there were those who associated practice nursing with the opportunity to develop a definite nursing career. Six nurses took this view and believed practice nursing offered a positive career choice. These responses were more common among those recently appointed to practice nurse posts, newly qualified nurses and those who worked full time. These nurses felt, for instance, that practice nursing was on a par with district nursing and health visiting. They consequently made the conscious decision to be a practice nurse.

When asked about their reasons for remaining a practice nurse, different aspirations became evident. Again, these aspirations provide an insight into the aspects of their work that become important to practice nurses and ones they are likely to protect. Two practice nurses explicitly viewed their work as a vocation. This small proportion is perhaps surprising given that the idea of vocation is embedded in many accepted practices and attitudes in nursing. It was more common, however, for the practice nurses included in this study to accept some assumptions of vocation in nursing. Most nurses, for example, often said it is the patients who made the job or that they liked helping and looking after people. They did not, however, identify themselves as having a particular vocation. Thus the idea of vocation, although acknowledged in their work, did not explain their decision to remain a practice nurse.

The more common response, expressed by 37 respondents, was to see practice nursing as a career. These nurses were committed to the professional development and establishment of practice nursing. This response included those who pursued practice nursing as a definite career, those dissatisfied with their previous nursing employment and those wishing to combine caring for a family with nursing employment. For those who entered practice nursing because of dissatisfaction with their previous nursing employment, the career opportunities of practice nursing only became apparent after they had taken up their post. A practice nurse said:

> *I thought I would try practice nursing. I didn't expect to enjoy it ... I thought it [practice nursing] was a backwater. But my eyes have been opened now. I didn't come in to practice nursing with high expectations. I thought after a few months I would be bored and go back to hospital. I didn't.*

Once these nurses entered practice nursing they soon became committed to the development of practice nursing and sought to establish its professional status. There was one practice nurse who sought a well-paid career whether in nursing or elsewhere. If she became dissatisfied with practice nursing she said she would move on to another job. Sixteen nurses regarded practice nursing simply as a job. Issues such as professional development, involvement in the practice or continuing training and education were of less interest to them. Nurses adopting this view were more likely to be family centred, work part time and to be less concerned about a career in nursing.

The nature and pattern of practice nursing

As we have seen, practice nursing is characterized by a range of activities undertaken in the practice and the patient's home: treatment room tasks; chronic disease management; health promotion; family planning; counselling and advice; and health assessments. The empirical accounts confirmed this and suggested that three general features characterize the nurse's role. First, there was no one task that predominated in their work and practice nurses valued this variety. Second, practice nurses agreed that there was more to their work than the simple completion of the immediate task. One remarked:

> *Often they come in here for something simple ... But it's just an excuse. You ask how they are and the floodgates open.*

Practice nurses were particularly keen to emphasize the wider implications of their work as many felt that practice nursing had an unfair reputation for being task orientated. This, they felt, undermined the professional credibility of practice nursing. Third, there was no particular type of work that a practice nurse consistently refused to do; it depended on specific circumstances and the nurse's perception of her competence.

According to the practice nurses the broad range of work performed by them is assumed with varying degrees of responsibility and included: offering support activities for GPs; performing delegated clinical activities requiring competence and skill; and undertaking work requiring independent judgement and action. GPs, for their part, still regarded treatment room tasks as fundamental to the work of practice nurses. Other work valued by GPs included health promotion, chronic disease management and family planning. GPs would use practice nurses for 'one-off' home visits, such as health assessments of people over 75, or when they experienced difficulties in delegating work, such as venepuncture, to the community nursing service.

The organization of work

Most practice nurses felt they had considerable autonomy in organizing their work. GPs usually issued general guidelines, leaving the practice nurse to work out the specific detail. This gave the practice nurse flexibility to develop her role and specialize in areas that interested her. Referrals, although accepted from a variety of sources, were largely initiated by the GP. Beyond this, GPs have little day-to-day interest in organizing the activities of practice nurses, thereby allowing them considerable autonomy in their work.

Practice nurses' experience of supervision in general practice was largely managerial and concerned with ensuring that the policy and procedures of the practice were followed. Clinical supervision, however, was rarely clarified and the overall experience of practice nurses suggested they worked to ad hoc and informal models. One nurse remarked:

I expect the GP doesn't know what I do most of the time.

Perhaps because of this, practice nurses felt accountable to the UKCC professional code of conduct. Occasionally this involved refusing to undertake delegated tasks if the nurse felt it was not part of her work or outside her competence. One said:

I mean it's up to me. I'm accountable for what I do. I would happily say, 'I'm sorry I'm not doing that'.

GPs also emphasized the importance of managerial forms of supervision and identified protocols as central to this supervisory relationship. GPs, however, had a limited understanding of both the nature and scope of a nurse's professional responsibility.

For most practice nurses their immediate and practical experience of team working was derived from working with other practice nurses. The wider community nursing team, including district nurses and health visitors, had less relevance for practice nurses. Of those practice nurses who worked together, most operated according to some notion of skill mix. However, this rarely involved an absolute and clear delineation of role. Some GPs felt there was a cohesive primary health-care team made up of practice nurses and community nurses, while others felt there was a division between their practice nurses and other community nurses. In the future GPs would like greater control over the community nursing service. They would also like to see less emphasis placed on the current distinctions among practice nurses, district nurses and health visitors.

Training and education

The contrast between practice nursing and their previous employment convinced many nurses of the relevance of induction courses. Practice nurses remarked that an induction course combining training in basic tasks, such as taking blood, with a more general programme on the role of the practice nurse in primary health care would be particularly useful. Few, however, had experienced the benefit of such a course. Continuing education and training was a fundamental concern. Practice nurses, however, drew an important distinction between training and education. Training was seen as task specific, whereas education was associated with general professional development. Most nurses remarked that training rather than education dominated their working lives and this was seen as a practical response to working in general practice.

Most practice nurses did not face restricted training opportunities and they exercised considerable autonomy in the study days they attended. No practice operated a formal appraisal scheme which identified a nurse's training needs. The lack of formal agreed criteria in securing training and education had, however, begun to concern some practice nurses. Lack of future funds was identified as a potential problem, especially since GPs and FHSAs were perceived as becoming more aware of costs. Several nurses were critical about the content of formal study days and National Nursing Board courses and questioned their relevance to practice nursing. Ideally, nearly all practice nurses agreed it was necessary to have a recognized practice nurse qualification validated by the UKCC.

GPs usually delegate the issue of nurse training to the senior nurse or practice manager. Few GPs thought strategically about the types of training their nurses ought to pursue. Short study courses directly relevant to work the nurse performed in the practice were a priority for GPs. No GP specifically distinguished between education and training and few saw the importance of formal and systematic induction.

As we have seen, FHSAs have an extended role in primary health care and employed nurse advisers to support nurses. The role of these advisers covered three key functions: administrative; offering professional support and advice; and ensuring opportunities for education and training. Advisers were clear that their role was one of supporting, rather than managing, primary health care. One said:

> *We advise. That is the basis of our credibility. We must be sensitive to GPs being independent contractors.*

Nonetheless, FHSAs interpret the scope of their role differently and a continuum of their involvement emerged. At one extreme there are those FHSAs which have minimal involvement and take little interest in practice nursing, believing it to be the responsibility of the employing GP. At the other end of the scale are those FHSAs which take a more proactive interest and directly intervene, by attempting to target their budgets to ensure a more equitable distribution of the practice nurse resource. The more usual pattern is a mix of these two extremes. More generally, FHSA advisers felt that they had an important role in identifying and providing courses to meet practice nurses' educational and training needs. FHSA advisers agreed with the practice nurse view about the task-orientated nature of many courses and would have liked professional development to be given more emphasis. Few advisers thought it necessary to specify set numbers of study days each year for practice nurses, preferring training to be decided on the basis of need. Particular problems, such as funding, did emerge. Another difficulty was the individual nature of many nurses' training needs which made it difficult to organize a coherent training programme.

The role of health commissioners and NHS trusts

Health commissioners felt treatment room tasks, health promotion and chronic disease management represented the core responsibilities of practice nurses. Beyond this, most thought the practice nurse role was ill defined and imprecise and felt unable to evaluate the contribution of practice nursing to primary health care when commissioning community nursing services. One commissioning manager remarked:

> *We need to look at the whole primary health care team and look at the whole nursing resource in relation to the practice population ... Sometimes it does feel a bit chaotic.*

Commissioners, however, acknowledged the importance of practice nurses in primary health care, especially remarking on the benefits practice nursing brought for the patient. All commissioners planned to develop a more strategic and sophisticated vision of primary health-care commissioning that utilized the nursing resource in accordance with the needs of the local population. Incorporating practice nursing into the commissioning strategy was seen as fundamental to its eventual success.

NHS trust managers largely shared the commissioners' view of practice nursing, identifying treatment room tasks, chronic disease management and health promotion as the core responsibilities. Particular advantages of practice nursing included their ability to perform tasks in the practice without the patient having to wait and being more approachable than GPs. Nonetheless, most providers, whilst recognizing the importance of practice nurses to primary health care, emphasized that practice nursing was largely task orientated and unable to offer the specialist skills of district nursing or health visiting. One community nurse manager remarked:

> *Practice nurses are very task orientated. District nurses have three years training and a much broader holistic view. They're more aware of things available from other services. I'm not sure practice nurses are.*

The primary focus of an NHS community trust was developing a community nursing service based on the principles of quality and efficiency. Providers perceived the development of practice nursing as being marginal to this, since this was outside their direct managerial control. Indeed, most providers, although emphasizing the importance of teamworking, felt that practice nurses represented a potential source of competition and threat to the services they provided.

The future of practice nursing

GPs and practice nurses expressed specific hopes and ambitions for the development of practice nursing. GPs, as we shall see, stressed the importance of nursing role development to meet *their* general medical service responsibilities. Practice nurses, on the other hand, emphasized the importance of professional development.

GPs regarded practice nursing as central to the future success of primary health care and most envisaged developing the practice nurse role. From their accounts three different options became apparent: increasing the responsibility of practice nurses; introducing prescribing rights for practice nurses; and developing the nurse practitioner role. Two-thirds of GPs saw practice nurses as able to develop their present flexibility by taking on greater responsibility and achieving greater specialization. Many of these GPs, for example, believed that in the future practice nurses would specialize in specific aspects of primary health care. Nevertheless, many GPs felt there were definite limits to the development of practice nursing; for instance, most felt that nurses should not be involved in diagnosis.

GPs, however, had more mixed views about nurse prescribing. The issue of developing nurse prescribing has been raised in several policy documents and the situation has been clarified with the announcement of pilot nurse-prescribing sites (see Chapter 4). Nevertheless, the demonstration sites only give opportunities to those nurses working in fundholding practices who hold either a district nurse or health visitor qualification. Involvement of practice nurses in these developments, therefore, would seem limited. However, remarks from many of the GPs suggest that practice nurses do have some influence on the prescribing process. In some cases practice nurses can even be said to be 'prescribing'. Two GPs, for example, gave out presigned scripts to nurses to use for minor conditions. A further five GPs would sign scripts made out by the practice nurses.

Practice nurses' accounts confirmed the nurse's influence on prescribing. More generally, nine of the GPs interviewed remarked on the advantages of giving limited prescribing rights to practice nurses. One fundholding GP remarked:

> *Prescribing would be useful. As things stand at the moment the nurse runs the asthma clinic and she's got a protocol and she might think a child is not well controlled on ventilin. And she may want to give it something else. She would have to write the prescription and I'd have to sign it … It wastes both our time.*

All GPs in favour of nurse prescribing, however, emphasized the importance of clearly defined prescribing rights, such as prescribing within specified areas, perhaps from a limited list. Most of these GPs also stressed the importance of the nurse working within set protocols and obtaining appropriate training. Practice nurses largely accepted this.

Developing the nurse practitioner role was a less common suggestion among those GPs interviewed. A third of the sample expressed definite enthusiasm for the idea. Definitions of a nurse practitioner, however, varied greatly among these GPs. As with prescribing, the nurse practitioner was viewed with caution by many GPs, even those who expressed interest in the idea. One fundholding GP questioned whether it was possible to have a third role in between that of GP and practice nurse. Other GPs were unsure about the control they could exercise over a more autonomous practitioner. This comment was typical:

> *The nurse practitioner? I'm not sure. I prefer attached staff. You can't have people uncoordinated or meddling in the community.*

More generally, GPs were happy to develop the work of the practice nurse but in a way that did not threaten their own role. They still wanted some control over the services offered by general practice and, more specifically, wanted to maintain the professional distinction between doctors and nurses. Allowing nurses to diagnose, prescribe or adopt a nurse practitioner role, for example, would threaten this distinction. Most GPs, therefore, were happy to develop the practice nurse role but only under conditions they could specify.

Nearly all the nurses interviewed expected to remain as practice nurses because they believed the profession was of considerable value to primary health care. In emphasizing their value to primary health care, practice nurses are supported by the views of their employing GP. This consensus forms the basis of possible alliances between GPs and practice nurses, especially if the present working arrangement were threatened by others such as NHS trust managers, health commissioners or the Department of Health. When specifically discussing their future role, practice nurses tended to focus on increasing their professional status: the greater professional status they could achieve, the greater their opportunity to exercise discretion. Within this context, a third of practice nurses interviewed expressed definite ideas of how they wished to progress. This usually involved increasing specialization in areas such as chronic disease management and family planning. Several wished to acquire formal training and educational qualifications to maintain their professional identity. For similar reasons, two-thirds of nurses held aspirations of becoming a nurse practitioner, although again there was no agreed definition of what the role entailed. Five nurses, however, felt that practice nursing offered no future for them. Two of these had been in practice nursing for some time and felt they were too old to develop their role further. The other three nurses felt they could not progress any further in practice nursing and were uncertain what else they could do.

Twenty-eight of the nurses interviewed in this study, and this included those confident about their own future, expressed some disquiet about the general future of practice nursing. For most practice nurses this remained a potential rather than real threat. Nevertheless, practice nurses perceived an increasing 'managerialism' in primary health care, which they felt was detrimental to their professional role. One nurse said:

> You're independent. You work on your own and manage your own time. But I can see that changing. There is tighter and tighter control. We're going back to an unhappy environment.

Seven nurses, for example, commented specifically that increasing administration meant they had less time to spend with patients. This tension is common to other forms of nursing, with management and administration seen as undermining the fulfilment of professional obligations (McKay 1990). However, because many nurses entered practice nursing due to dissatisfaction with their previous nursing post, the threat of increasing 'managerialism' assumes a special significance. Practice nurses would attempt to avoid increasing managerial control; after all, this was the reason many nurses left their previous employment.

Before leaving this discussion about the future of practice nursing, it is important to discuss the concerns expressed by other health-care agencies about the growth in practice nurse numbers. The key issue is who has control over practice nursing; concerns which could have a bearing on the development of practice nursing. At present, the GP employment and management of practice nurses is supported by government policy. Health commissioners and provider units, however, can challenge some aspects of the GPs' role and specifically question their ability to employ practice nurses.

Representatives from purchasing agencies and community nursing units criticized the *ad hoc* development of practice nursing. In particular, all commissioning agencies believed considerable inequalities in the distribution of the practice nurse resource existed, because posts were originally allocated according to the demands of general practice rather than notions of patient need. To this extent, commissioning authorities were more concerned to establish an equitable distribution of resources organized according to a sense of priorities rather than universal need. Community nurse providers, on the other hand, voiced concerns that the perceived lack of a clearly defined role accompanying this growth in practice nurse numbers created the potential for role overlap and duplication with other community nurses.

CONCLUSION

This chapter has evaluated the emergence and development of practice nursing from the perspectives of the different stakeholders within a pluralistic theoretical and empirical framework. Evaluating the emergence and development of practice nursing is not simply of historical interest but raises fundamental issues that will influence the future development of practice nursing and primary health care. To this extent, the tensions generated by the different interests of the stakeholders – practice nurses, GPs, trust managers, health commissioners, representatives of the NHS Executive and Department of Health – and the subsequent organizational and policy initiatives that emerge provide the context in which practice nursing will develop.

As we have seen, practice nurses represent a substantial primary health-care nursing resource. Developments in health-care policy created the major demand for nurses in general practice. The introduction of the 1990 GP contract and the system of financial incentives associated with it were fundamental to these developments. An initial lack of financial restrictions, sanctioned by the Department of Health, and the FHSAs' ability to utilize these meant that funding for these nursing posts was readily available.

GPs felt community nurses would have difficulty in meeting their new responsibilities and were attracted to the idea of directly employing a nurse to meet the targets specified in the 1990 GP contract. Once the potential for practice nursing had been established, nurses found it an attractive job option. It offered autonomy, flexible, often part-time work, with opportunities for high levels of patient contact. Most nurses, in striving to maintain a sense of career, were committed to sustaining the professional status of practice nursing. When discussing their own future role, for example, practice nurses tended to emphasize those elements of role development that increased their professional status. Practice nurses would especially resist increasing managerial control over their work, particularly since this was the reason many nurses left their previous employment. Locality commissioners and managers of community nursing trusts expressed concerns about the sudden growth in practice nurse numbers. The key issue was who had control over the practice nursing resource. At present the GP employment and management of practice nurses is supported by government policy. However, purchasing agencies and provider units can begin to challenge the present relationship between the GP and practice nurse.

More generally, the possible influence of the community trust and health commissioner reminds us that the debate about practice nursing is wider than practice nursing per se and could raise broader issues about the organization of primary health care. Current policies on community health and social care, and in particular the changing balance between primary and secondary care, will bring continuing pressures for extending the practice nurse's role (Marsh & Dawes 1995). The restructuring of the NHS, however, raises more general questions about the range, quality, organization and effectiveness of primary health-care services (Department of Health 1996a,b). In particular, there are moves to encourage a more systematic pooling of primary health-care nursing resources to take account of the needs of the population they serve (Department of Health 1996b)

Consequently, those involved in primary health care are having to examine their roles, responsibilities and aims. The development of primary health care does not occur within a vacuum and is informed by previous practice, interests and policy initiatives. The evaluation offered by this chapter identifies the policy and practice tensions that will inform the future of practice nursing: first, the impact of changing role, intensification of skill mix and the need for an adequately trained nursing workforce on practice nursing; second, between the GPs' aspirations to continue to develop the service they value and the health commissioner's wish to ensure a more appropriate and effective use of the practice nurse resource; third, between the nurses' sense of flexibility and autonomy and the demands to develop a more managed primary-care system; and finally between practice nurses' aspirations to be recognized as a professional specialization and GPs' continuing, task-specific expectations.

QUESTIONS FOR DISCUSSION

◆ What implications does locality commissioning have for practice nursing?

◆ To what extent is practice nursing an emerging profession?

◆ Do practice nurses have adequate professional support?

◆ What is the likely relationship between practice nurses and general practitioners?

◆ How can practice nurses best work with other community nurses as part of a primary health-care team?

ANNOTATED BIBLIOGRAPHY

Atkin K, Lunt N, Parker G, Hirst M 1993 Nurses count: a national census of practice nurses. Social Policy Research Unit, University of York
Atkin K, Lunt N 1995 Nurses in practice: the role of practice nursing in primary health care. Social Policy Research Unit, University of York

Two reports describing the first national census of practice nursing in England and Wales and a more indepth qualitative evaluation of their work in primary health care. Together, the two reports provide a comprehensive and empirically based discussion of practice nursing. The first provides a national profile of practice nurses, presenting data on the work they undertake, their professional training and experiences and their training needs, and discusses the implications of these findings for primary health care. The second presents a more detailed view of practice nursing as seen by the nurses themselves, by the general practitioners who employ them and by those who have responsibility for managing, planning and delivering community nursing services.

Damant M, Martin C, Openshaw S 1994 Practice nursing: stability and change. Mosby, London

One of the few substantial accounts of practice nursing, considering past trends, current themes and future developments. The book is strong in all three areas and is a useful read for anyone with an interest in practice nursing.

Audit Commission 1993 Practice makes perfect: the role of the family health service authority. HMSO, London

This report – in a section written by Barbara Stilwell – provides a detailed statistical account of the work of practice nurses. The nature of the study – a sample rather than a census of practice nurses – means it provides more detail than Nurses Count. *The rest of the report, although dated, still provides a good introduction to the management of primary health care.*

REFERENCES

Atkin K, Hirst M 1994 Costing practice nurses: implications for primary health care. Discussion paper series 117. Centre for Health Economics, University of York

Atkin K, Lunt N 1996a Negotiating the role of the practice nurse in general practice. Journal of Advanced Nursing 24: 498–505

Atkin K, Lunt N 1996b The role of the practice nurse in primary health care: managing and supervising the practice nurse resource. Journal of Nursing Management 4: 85–92

Atkin K, Lunt N, Parker G, Hirst M 1993 Nurses count: a national census of practice nurses. Social Policy Research Unit, University of York

Audit Commission 1993 Practice makes perfect: the role of the family health service authority. HMSO, London

Bourdieu P 1994 Distinction: a social critique of taste. Routledge, London

Damant M, Martin C, Openshaw S 1994 Practice nursing: stability and change. Mosby, London

Department of Health 1996a Primary care; delivering the future. The Stationery Office, London

Department of Health 1996b Choice and opportunity: primary care – the future. The Stationery Office, London

Goldberg E M, Connelly N 1982 The effectiveness of social care of the elderly: an overview of recent and current evaluative research. Heinemann, London

Guba E G, Lincoln Y S 1989 Fourth generation evaluation. Sage, London

Gubrium J F, Silverman D 1989 The politics of field research: sociology beyond enlightenment. Sage, London

Hammersley M, Atkinson P 1983 Ethnography: principles in practice. Tavistock, London

Hirst M, Atkin K, Lunt N 1994 Variations in practice nursing: implications for family health service authorities. Health and social care in the community 3: 89–97

Hirst M, Atkin K, Lunt N 1998 Distribution of practice nurses in England and Wales. Journal of health services research and policy 3: 131–138

Hoggett P 1991 Modernisation, political strategy and the welfare state: an organisational perspective. School For Advanced Urban Studies, Bristol

Levick P 1992 The Janus face of community care legislation: an opportunity for radical possibilities? Critical social policy 12 (1): 75–92

Lightfoot J, Baldwin S, Wright K 1992 Nursing by numbers? Setting staffing levels for district nursing and health visiting services. Social Policy Research Unit and Centre for Health Economics, University of York

McKay L 1990 Nursing: just another job? In: Abbott P, Wallace C (eds) The sociology of the caring professions. Falmer, Basingstoke

Marsh G N, Dawes M L 1995 Establishing a minor illness nurse in a busy practice. British Medical Journal 310: 21–31

Martin C 1992 Attached, detached, or new recruits? British Medical Journal 305: 348–350

Merton R K, Kendall P L 1946 The focused interview. American Journal of Sociology 51: 541–557

Mishler E G 1986 Research interviewing: context and narrative. Harvard University Press, Cambridge

NHS Management Executive 1993 Nursing in primary health care: new world, new opportunities. HMSO, London

Outhwaite W 1975 Understanding social life: the method called Verstehen. George Allen and Unwin, London

Poulton B C, West M A 1993a Primary health care team effectiveness: developing a constituency approach. Health and Social Care in the Community 2: 77–84

Poulton B C, West M A 1993b Effective multidisciplinary teamwork in primary health care. Journal of Advanced Nursing 18: 918–925

Reedy B L E C, Phillips P R, Newell D J 1976 Nurses and nursing in primary medical care in England. British Medical Journal 2: 1304–1306

Robinson G 1990 The future for practice nurses. British Journal of Medical Practice April: 132–133

Robinson G, Beaton S, White P 1993 Attitudes towards practice nurses – survey of a sample of general practitioners in England and Wales. British Journal of Medical Practice 43: 25–29

Ross F 1991 The screening debate. Nursing Times 87 (26): 59–61

Ross F, Bower P, Sibbald B 1994 Practice nurses: characteristics, workload and training needs. British Journal of General Practice 44: 15–18

Selby A, Winkler F, Brown P 1992 More practice. Health service journal 19 March: 31

Smith G, Cantley C 1985 Assessing health care: a study in organisational evaluation. Open University Press, Milton Keynes

Statutory Instruments 1990 No. 1330 (6), Family health service authorities. HMSO, London

Stilwell B 1988 Origins and development of the role. In: Bowling A, Stilwell B (eds) The nurse in family practice. Scutari Press, London

Twigg J, Atkin K 1994 Carers perceived: policy and practice in informal care. Open University Press, Buckingham

8

Evaluating learning disability – embracing change

Tony Thompson   Peter Mathias

KEY ISSUES

- ◆ Organizational and professional defences tend to resist changes with the potential to benefit people with a disability.

- ◆ The means by which individuals and organizations attempt to minimize anxiety are often associated with change through a process of denial.

- ◆ The nursing establishment, and its inherent traditionalism, act as a means of clinging to the past and appealing to history or past authority in order to justify the status quo.

- ◆ Policies and procedures are often sanctioned by nursing organizations in ways which ensure they become self-sustaining.

- ◆ The concept of 'supersimplification' (Toffler 1970) is often a feature of service delivery, structure and policy. Services often seek unitary solutions to highly complex problems, e.g. normalization, programming, challenging behaviour statements.

INTRODUCTION

This chapter presents the underlying principles and components of an effective and integrated community-based service for people with a learning disability. Further, obstacles to the development of such services are identified and the values which lie behind them outlined. The chapter points to the need for a shift from outmoded and inappropriate services towards models which reflect the value of individuals with a learning disability to society as a whole. The evidence for this argument is grounded in the disciplines of education, law, social work, psychology, medicine and politics. The arguments presented also reflect the need to recognize the lack of consensus surrounding the rationale for, and consequences of, change in the arena of practical care for those people with a learning disability.

The chapter focuses on issues of service structure and policy but does so with reference to conflicting discourses on the delivery of efficient service systems. Interprofessional education is a developing, albeit sometimes implicit, theme in many of these discourses. As such, the reader is requested to consider how the philosophies and goals underpinning emerging services for learning disabled people are affected by the interaction of the competing discourses of the various groups involved at service level.

Attention is drawn to the need for evaluation based upon answers to key questions which relate to professional responsibility. For example: how can the community practitioner create, design and establish structures that allocate clear responsibility for providing community services, including monitoring and accountability mechanisms?

The chapter also places recent policy initiatives with a significant impact on the learning disability branch of nursing (such as the Chief Nursing Officers' consensus conference and the Department of Health's document 'Continuing the commitment') in the 'real-world' context of service delivery. These services are examined from a perspective which recognizes the need to balance quantity and quality on an ongoing and coordinated basis.

THE PROFESSIONAL PREREQUISITE

The widening of the concept of disability and the need for disabled people to be empowered in the shaping of their own future, together with the emergence of a plurality of service provision, demand increased input from a wider group of professions than was available a decade ago. The nature of care within the community has sometimes increased the divisions of interests, responsibility and authority between employers, professional associations, trade unions, educational authorities and representatives of service users or 'consumers'.

A particular example of this is the expectation that those nurses working to the UKCC Code of Conduct (UKCC 1992) will act in such a manner as to justify public trust and confidence, to uphold and enhance the good standing and reputation of the profession and to serve the public interest and interest of patients and clients. Such bold aspirations can conflict with the professional's wish to promote and safeguard the well-being of their clients by utilizing the media to raise public awareness when working within employment conditions which effectively 'gag' organizational dissent.

THE HISTORICAL DIMENSION

Contemporary themes, conflicts and concerns are perhaps best viewed through the conceptual lens of history and its relationship with disabled people. Early history points to the 'synergy' between services caring for the disabled and early professional structures. Most practitioners are well aware of the treatment of people with a disability in the past and the lack of specialism surrounding it. Individuals were often confined to institutions associated with insanity and very often received the same treatment modalities regardless of need. These modalities were diverse and often rooted in mythology.

We know that in early primitive and nomadic tribes women often provided care for those that were sick on the encampment and that disease and illnesses were associated with evil spirits and supernatural phenomena. Perhaps it was not surprising that those seen as 'non-contributors' to society were abandoned. In that era there is little evidence to suggest any organized arrangements for protection of the person who was deemed handicapped. Later, when churches or temples of the Egyptian influence focused upon holistic healing, rudimentary nursing care for the sick became apparent. The Egyptians and the Greeks provided, within this historical context, humane and remedial care for those considered to be insane. Prior to this, the Spartans, Greeks and Romans abandoned or sacrificed defective children. Wealthy Romans sometimes took the atypical step of maintaining the retarded person in their own domestic fold to act as a type of jester to entertain visiting guests. Slaves were seen as being appropriate to care for such people considered to be incurable or insane.

The early Christian era brought new changes, mainly through the concept of charity and its association with a variety of religious orders. By the Middle Ages a more punitive approach to those people thought to be possessed by supernatural beings was prevalent. It was not until the Sisters of Charity, based in the Paris asylum of the Bice Tré, that humane understanding became a feature of professional care. England had to wait until the era of King Henry VIII for hospitals to be organized and financially underwritten, thereby ensuring the provision of state-sponsored care for disabled people.

During the 17th century the mentally ill and criminals were often incarcerated together. It was not until the Bethlem Royal Hospital purposely separated criminals from the insane kept in the asylum that any real organization of directed care took place. However, care during that era was also associated with terribly impoverished conditions. Patients were often infected and infested with disease and parasites. Rudimentary and cruel practices were prevalent but despite this, the idea of professional 'care' began to develop.

Nursing and caring for people with a disability have followed similar, cyclical paths. They were both abandoned by the ancients, received humane treatments during the era of Christianity and persecuted during the

Reformation. The one consistent factor has been that throughout all periods of the cycle, the disabled person has often been viewed as an object of entertainment and derision.

In the latter part of the 19th century care continued to be organized along categorical lines. Distinctions were made between the severity of handicapping conditions and these were reflected in service terminology. Categories such as idiots and imbeciles emerged as the primary means of identifying the disabled. Doctors continued to categorize handicap by organic or physiological anomalies and services started to be grouped according to the likelihood of effectiveness of input. Therapeutic methods continued to be based in institutions, primarily as public opinion viewed those deemed to be mentally retarded as a threat to the community. However, the organization of colonies of institutional care evolved with the intention of reflecting better and more normal living and working conditions. The concept of the colony enabled supervised care but also allowed for economic contributions from the disabled in the form of remuneration for work associated with simple tasks in agricultural or domestic environments.

By the early 20th century education began to be a major feature in the care of the disabled. And whilst the community were generally ill at ease with people with mentally handicapping conditions, special education developed and new opportunities for such development were recognized. In the latter part of the 20th century changes in both nursing and the field of learning disability have advanced the notion of specialty preparation in order that services can be expanded and further organized. The philosophy of care has gradually moved from that of custody towards supportive caring in the general community. Provision now involves the efforts of central and local government, unpaid carers and professionals.

Throughout these changes, nursing influence has developed. In the United Kingdom a chief nursing officer (CNO) works at a senior level within the government. The specialty of learning disabilities is recognized by the CNO who has a nurse on her staff whose background is in learning disability. Nursing in an institutional sense has increasingly become a distinct and influential activity, whilst community learning disability nursing has developed its own specialty in the arena of community health. Nursing bodies, in order to better prepare nurses for such specialized activity, have formulated and designed various curricular and training programmes. Moreover, there has been increasing interdependence between nursing and other fields associated with learning disability, especially social work.

CONTEMPORARY SERVICE DEVELOPMENT

The 1990 NHS and Community Care Act introduced significant changes based on the recognition that health service and local authority agencies should work together. It became essential that clarification of strategic aims and intentions took place between those bodies, with particular regard to the sharing of responsibilities, objectives, criteria for assessment, commissioning intentions and the coordination of services aimed at improving the health of the nation. The emphasis upon the development of new service structures for long-term care, which was a theme during the 1980s, was reinforced. The deinstitutionalization of long-term care was paralleled by changes in the locus of activity associated with the provision of acute or secondary-care services.

Since April 1993, purchasing responsibilities for residential services have rested with local authority social services departments. This made hospital discharges to long-stay care dependent upon needs assessment by the local authority. Interagency dependence has therefore increased and collaboration is a necessary process if the intentions of the NHS and Community Care Act are to be realized. The breadth of collaboration now includes education, housing and leisure services. The principal elements of the implementation of the concept of community care include:

♦ empowering people to have a greater degree of influence over how they conduct their lives and the services that are needed in supporting them to do so;
♦ Aiming to provide the correct level of care and supporting structures to assist people in the achievement of maximum potential and independence, together with the acquisition of basic living skills to assist them in achieving such potential;
♦ enabling people to live as normal a life as possible in their own homes and environments or in scaled environments based upon acceptable domesticity.

The demands on services which meet these elements are obviously dependent upon the overall prevalence of disability. This in turn depends greatly upon the methodology used to estimate such prevalence. The total prevalence of severe learning disability making particular demands upon community resources has been estimated as being in the order of 3–4 people per 1000 population. However, differing mortality rates mean that as the population ages, the proportion with the greatest level of learning disability falls. All local authorities are expected to keep a register of people with a disability. A register-based study conducted by North West Thames Region has indicated that the rate is 3.7/3.8 per 1000 amongst the population aged between 15 and 44 years. Amongst 45–64-year-olds an actual prevalence rate of 2.4 per 1000 is projected and 1.25 per 1000 population aged over 65 (Farmer et al 1991).

ON POLICY DEVELOPMENT

The term 'community care' first rose to prominence during the 1970s with efforts to relocate and rehabilitate long-stay patients away from institutional care and towards that contained within the wider community. The way in which nursing services have responded to this development often reflects the confusion around a concept of community care which often appears as a description of services rather than as a statement of intended outcome.

It is only lately that central government community care policy has encouraged proactivity rather than taking a reactive stance to adverse conditions prevailing within institutional care. Goodwin (1989) argues that central policy appears to follow, rather than mould, professional opinion and preference. For example, the 1959 Mental Health Act sought to foster not community care for people with mental health problems but 'treatment in the community'. Such reformation was necessary to address the challenges arising as a result of changes in professional practice and political-economic theories, rather than constituting a reforming measure resulting from enlightened thinking. In other words, the community care policy on mental health issues only represented a response to the crisis associated with the care in long-stay institutions.

Bulmer (1987) offers four different types of use of the term 'community care', each of which has obvious implications for the ways in which nurses offer care in community environments (Box 8.1).

The definitions are quite useful for understanding the way in which different services contribute to the community care process. From the NHS perspective, the concept is often seen simply as one of getting people away from hospital care. Despite a number of government circulars and publications, the

---

Box 8.1 The disputed concept of community care

◆ An origin which was to be interpreted as delivering care away from large institutions, particularly those erected during the Victorian era.

◆ Delivery of a variety of professional services away from the major hospital resource, seen in areas such as community nursing and community mental health teams.

◆ It could be designated as care by the community, which would imply the involvement of voluntary agencies and families. The inequity of the informal care burden is addressed, though not necessarily resolved, by the NHS and Community Care Act of 1990.

◆ The term could be utilized to describe provision of care which was value based and in as ordinary a setting as possible.

'how' of doing this was often not clear. The 1971 White Paper on mental handicap services, for instance, included some vague strategy statements supporting the service user and their family, but of five main policy objectives, only one made recommendations for services actually within the community (Wistow 1985).

Policy sentiment reinforcing community care as service intent has existed for many years. It was not, however, supported by financial backing until the concept of joint finance entered the policy arena in the 1970s. Even here, though, there were so many restrictions imposed as to lead the House of Commons Social Services Committee to refer to underfinanced and under-staffed community care provision.

During this time nursing continued its 'synergistic' development with policy more generally. The revision of the nursing syllabus took place in 1982 and this became an influential document. It reflected the need to respond to the recommendations of the Jay Committee (Cmnd 7468), primarily that social service departments should be the lead organization in the training of community professionals. Jay also suggested the Social Work Council should become responsible for education and training, which were hitherto the realm of the General Nursing Council for England and Wales.

Following Jay, the highly critical 1986 report from the Audit Commission, 'Making a Reality of Community Care', indicated the anomalies and defects within a system dominated by perverse incentives, inaccurate targeting of resources and waste (Box 8.2).

The report helped provoke the government to commission Sir Roy Griffiths to review community care (1988). It was following this that the White Paper 'Caring for People' was published and the 1990 NHS and Community Care Act was formed.

Box 8.2 Making a reality of community care

◆ The inequity of the burden placed upon family carers, especially women.

◆ The heavy tapping of the social security revenue due to the fact that access to residential and nursing home care was to be made available without adequate assessment of care needs.

◆ The lack of capital planning for community-based alternatives to residential care.

◆ The lack of staff development opportunities for community-based alternatives to residential care.

◆ The lack of staff development opportunities for community care services which occurred at the same time as a tremendous increase in the hospital rundown.

The 1989 White Paper focused on the various aspects of the community care system and pointed to a history of weakness and neglect. An indicator of the urgency and the priority afforded to the project by government at that time was seen in the speed with which the 1989 NHS and Community Care Bill followed the White Paper and its subsequent implementation. The Act introduced radical change in health and social service provision on a scale not seen since the 1940s. Glynn & Perkins (1995) suggest that this reformation be viewed from four standpoints.

◆ **Shifting the balance between institutional and community care.** This was seen in the explicit encouragement of local authorities to shift the emphasis away from institutional in favour of domiciliary-based care. This was reflected in the strategic split between acute and community care in the health service. Therefore the separation of purchasers from providers in health should have a similar reflection in community social care provisions.

◆ **Development of supply-led versus needs-led care.** This strategic objective of central government policy can be seen to be highlighted in a variety of specific actions and is intended to move the community care system away from supply-led, provider-dominated services, which were seen to be a feature of postwar social policy, to a system of needs-led and policy-dominated services.

◆ **Pluralism.** This is seen in explicit and reinforced policy emphasis on the mixed economy of care. This particular effect has had ramifications for health service staff who may well have qualifications which are not uniformly sought or required by independent and voluntary providers of services. The divergent demographic and economic features indicated earlier in this chapter may well force even greater radical thoughts as to the degree of pluralism which we will see in the future. However, the shape of this pluralistic service context for practice will be shaped – indeed has been shaped – by the fact that the community care reforms reflect a number of features with the broader privatisation thrust of the Thatcher and Major governments, the legacy of which has only just begun to be addressed by the present habour government.

◆ **The shifting balance between NHS and local authority funding.** This last element of community care policy reflects the alteration in the balance of responsibility for decision making and funding between the NHS and local government. This has been achieved through the transfer of funds from the Department of Social Security to social services departments with the latter being given the lead role in the provision of community care services, the intention being improved collaboration and coordination in planning, commissioning and provision of services.

It is clear that responsibility for the provision of services cuts across a number of agencies. Because of this, the distinction between health and social care will never be clear cut. For instance, those departments that are responsible for implementing housing policy are often an important feature in the provision of services for people with a learning disability. Whilst each has an equally crucial role to play, there is often confusion and friction between agencies leading to a picture of resource gaps in total provision.

This context presents a particular challenge for those professionals that have the competence and qualifications for working within health and local authority services. This challenge revolves around the need to move beyond short-term goals towards implementation agendas based on longer term planning for accurately targeted community care services. So far, services appear to have done well on the rhetoric and less well on the action. Progress on interprofessional working has been patchy and extreme and true patient participation is a long way off.

Service managers in both health and social services have had to increase productivity and reduce costs. They are required to look closely at the costs and results achieved by the different services that they manage. Moreover, this context of cost consciousness has fostered a view which sees the continuance of the community nursing status quo as a result of policy-induced 'pragmatism'. Specifically, nursing services were purchased because they were most easily understood by referral agencies (DHAs and GP fundholders) and therefore easier to sell than the interdisciplinary and the interagency concept implied by more adventurous care solutions (Ovretveit et al 1997).

CONTEMPORARY STATEMENTS RELATING TO LEARNING DISABILITY NURSING PRACTICE

New practice and career pathways are emerging within learning disability services as a result of the move to prevent fragmentation of services. The interprofessional explorations of recent years have led to a flow of new skills, competences and knowledge. Learning disability nurses have found that it has proved useful to share ideas and practice and to become acquainted with new perspectives and approaches in order to be more effective in primary-care teams. Much more, however, is emerging – a body of practice which is habilitative and educational in both social and health senses, thus enabling and supporting people as they overcome difficulties in thinking, perception and emotion which have consequences for their participation in society. This changing practice base draws heavily on the principles of the social pedagogy movement described by Davies-Jones (1992).

The development of this thinking has been expounded by the authors and was further stimulated by the outcomes of the 1993 Department of Health-

---

Box 8.3 Opportunities for change – the five options

◆ Continuation of the learning disabilities branch within the family of nursing.

◆ Assimilation of prequalifying nurse training programmes for learning disability within the child, adult and mental health branches of Project 2000 and within a revised postqualifying framework.

◆ The emergence of a new profession, with contributions from social work, nursing and from informal carers specific to the care of people with learning disabilities.

◆ The concept of a new rehabilitation specialist with a focus on disability across a range of client groups.

◆ The assimilation of the RNMH programmes within the prequalifying social work curriculum.

---

sponsored conference 'Opportunities for Change: A New Direction for Nursing for People with Learning Disabilities'. Five options for change were put to the conference (Box 8.3).

Although option 1 prevailed as a central decision there was the strongest support in subsequent consultation for a combination of options 3, 4 and 5. The learning disability branch of nursing has been active in shaping initiatives which support this groundswell. They have coordinated activities within a range of agencies and professional groups to try and meet the complex needs of people with a learning disability. These efforts are particularly seen in the management of residential services. Nurses have long utilized best practice in enabling services to reflect domestic environments. However, in recent years increased emphasis has been placed on the empowerment of service users and carers through the application of the concept of advocacy.

Specialist nurses play an important role in promoting health gain in people with a learning disability. In order to pursue such gains, service values, costs and outcomes have to be considered. In doing so, learning disability nurses often find their contemporary practice is underpinned by a recognition that the concept of learning disability is far more than a singular 'medical' problem. The challenges to the delivery of services which learning disability nurses face are:

◆ they must help people with a learning disability to gain access to mainstream health and social-care provision;

◆ there must be provision of those specialist services that meet the complex needs of a person handicapped through having a learning disability.

In order to fully meet these needs, the disability nurse pursues three major aims:

- the maintenance and improvement of the 'total' health of people with learning disabilities;
- the creation of conditions which allow specialist interventions to reduce the cause of learning disability;
- the enhancement of the social support necessary for a person with a learning disability.

These aims test the interprofessional nature of service provision and can be seen to cluster around two areas: those that reflect specific health challenges (Box 8.4), and those which identify a wider, more holistic need for the disabled person (Box 8.5). Meeting these challenges requires a change in the culture of many services and practitioners.

PROFESSIONAL REACTION TO CHANGE

In the past three decades some individuals and organizations have responded

---

Box 8.4 The challenges relating to health in people with a learning disability

- Psychosocial health problems
- Mental health problems
- Behaviour that challenges the service
- Inadequate nutrition
- Epilepsy
- Communication problems
- Difficulty in mobilization
- Conditions of multiple sensory impairment

Box 8.5 General holistic needs of people with a learning disability

- The benefit of a family experience
- The right to dignity
- The right to respect
- The right to choice
- The pursuit of an independent life
- The design of integrated services
- Continuity and consistency of support

to the possibilities of the required change in negative ways. A typical response has been that of denial which is reflected in the view that some people are so disabled that they will always need institutional care. Traditionalism – that is, clinging to the past and appealing to history and past authority as justification for maintaining the status quo – has also been apparent. It is particularly so in those areas which specialize in care of people who challenge services and those who may present as a grave or immediate danger to themselves or others.

Allport, in his treatise of 1937, introduced the concept of functional autonomy. This theory holds that motives may become independent of their origins and continue to operate even though they are no longer functional. Thus, organizations that have been geared towards meeting the needs of the disabled person have often sanctified procedures and policies which are, in reality, redundant. The history of learning disability nursing is peppered with systems which have become self-sustaining in spite of inappropriateness.

Finally, the major defence of supersimplification (Toffler 1970), of seeking unitary solutions for highly complex problems, has sometimes enveloped current challenges, anticipated problems and unresolved issues. The best description of this in the field of learning disability has been in such terms introduced as panaceas for the challenges which change brings. For example, social role valorization, normalization, developmental programming and de-institutionalization all have the potential to be interpreted as singular, unitary solutions to the symptoms of service failure.

One vital aspect of evaluating the effect of these variables upon community services in the learning disability field is the concept of responsibility. Over a period of time only limited energy has been expended in the creation of robust structures which allocate clear accountability for provision of services. In reality this has meant that community services for learning disabled people have not developed to the necessary quantity and quality to meet client needs.

Some authorities have learnt from experience gained of the regulatory structures in place for nursing and residential homes and from the monitoring systems for meeting the special educational needs of disabled children. The type of evaluative procedures that are coming to the fore include environmental checking and inspection on a regular basis by professionals and service users who have been specifically trained to identify problems and develop corrective procedures. Another mechanism of evaluation includes setting up effective systems based on intermediate surveys by care providers for measuring their continuing needs, the offshoot being the development of continuing professional or in-service development. A third system is that of sanctioned or reinforced standards. Of course, these are just one dimension of implementing effective evaluative systems. Another particular focus is concerned with programming, a mechanism developed more widely in the United

States. This programme concentrates on whether there has been progress associated with the disabled person's attainment of skills.

Effective evaluation requires that mechanisms have to be in place that are a component of or are closely aligned to the care system that has been monitored. Amongst the most effective of these are those which require each community service provider to have a management board including representatives from a broad spectrum of interests, particularly service user groups. Accurate representation is critical because the organizational experience and knowledge of services can be a powerful arrangement to counter the weaknesses found within community systems. The advocacy movement has also been influential in promoting evaluation geared towards matching the personal needs of disabled people with the provisions of the service. This can be an effective tool for monitoring and reinforcing standards that are applicable to that service. These developments have to be contrasted with some of the constraining elements of evaluation found in traditional services. These revolve around the inertia found in large and complex organizations, together with bureaucracy, remote policy formation, multitudinous procedures, budget constraints and vague regulations. Altering this process has often meant seeking the approval of numerous people with vested interests, including those responsible for protecting professions and officials of a particular political persuasion who can affect the legislation surrounding disability services.

CONCLUSION

In order to change complex systems and therefore subject them to evaluative procedures, planners have to be prepared to unravel many complicated issues, particularly in the case of subcultures. Any evaluation of community services is usually affected by the retention of institutional arrangements for care. This source of resistance has been accurately recorded by Roos et al (1980).

◆ It would be economically unsound to sacrifice existing capital investment typically committed to large facilities – the big buildings, the land and renovations.
◆ The cost-benefit data comparing institutions with community-based residential programmes are still unclear and inconsistent.
◆ The funding streams currently available tend to favour institutions. Indeed, some of the programmes serve as disincentives to deinstitutionalization.
◆ Another major problem is the relative inaccessibility of services in community settings.
◆ Concern has also been expressed that community settings may lead to ineffective and inefficient deployment of resources.
◆ Since many administrators prefer management through control rather

than management through persuasion, decentralized community models provide an uncomfortable situation.

◆ Executives contend that it is much more difficult to clearly identify the focus of responsibility and accountability in a dispersed system than in a traditional, centralized model, such as a typical institution.

Such resistance to community-based services is not always the fault of the professional administrator; indeed, some parental and carer groups are questioning or resisting the notion of deinstitutionalization. These feelings cannot be dismissed as manifestations of overprotectiveness and their reasons can be based on realistic considerations (Twigg & Atkin 1994). In evaluative terms, the fears expressed revolve around the question of security of funding and the fact that community programmes can be tenuous and transitory.

Because the locus of responsibility is sometimes vague and confusing in community-based residential systems, parents may not know who to turn to when they wish to question or challenge the system. Concern may be raised about the health and safety aspects of some community facilities in that they may represent greater risks than the relatively self-contained institutional model of care. There is also the underlying anxiety that the move to community care can ultimately result in having children returned to parents who may feel unable or unwilling to cope with such a possibility. Only limited work has been undertaken on monitoring and evaluating the effects of such fears on parents who do not wish to reexperience past traumas or face the possibility that difficult decisions made in the past may not have been in their child's best interest.

All these concerns make evaluation absolutely essential in relation to decision processes about the types of community services made available to people with a learning disability, together with the need for responsible assessments which will more accurately identify the true needs of individuals who are actually dependent upon others. Bennis et al (1976) identified a real weakness in the decision-making process that yields outcomes based upon the identification of needs. Typically, when confronted with the problem of evaluation, decision makers tend to review available facts, decide to accept them at the moment, proceed with the decision process and present the solutions that more often than not are based upon their interpretation of a particular person's needs. In effect, they and the quality of their decisions are accountable only to themselves, since their claim to represent an individual in the decision space rests upon their interpretation of that person's needs as they relate to the system in general and not necessarily to the person in question. It is for this reason that decisions made about learning disabled people become more important due to the 'how' factor of 'why' they are made. Evaluators of the effectiveness of community systems may well find it useful to follow the criteria identified by Wolfensberger (1972) who cites the following features:

◆ programmes for individuals with a disability should be dispersed throughout the larger community as much as possible;
◆ services for individuals with a disability should be specialized enough to meet unique configurations of individual needs;
◆ services for citizens with a disability should be integrated into comparable services for the non-handicapped population to the greatest extent possible;
◆ the system must provide continuity in both interagency and intraagency functions.

If such assessment of a person's life in relation to community contact is to be made, this should be seen in the light of their unique traits and behaviours and the way in which they can make a valued contribution to their life's environment.

QUESTIONS FOR DISCUSSION

◆ How might a service management team devise a framework for evaluation which is both usable and yet reflects the complex nature of many learning disabled people's lives?
◆ What innovative national-level evaluatory frameworks have you encountered which could be translated into local frameworks for action?
◆ How might you go about addressing the moral requirement to involve service users in defining an evaluation's frame of reference?

ANNOTATED BIBLIOGRAPHY

Bingley W 1987 The mentally handicapped person as citizen. In: Alves E (ed) Mental handicap and the law. BPS, London

This makes a well-argued case for legal reform, identifying two particular deficiencies. First, in public law, the need to protect vulnerable people from neglect and abuse and second, in private law, resolving disputes and uncertainties of people with disabilities about their care.

Braddock D, Heller T 1985 the closure of mental handicap institutions. Trends in United States Mental Retardation 23 (4): 168–176

This offers a valuable comparative debate aligned with similar ventures in the UK. Based on criteria and definitions for evaluating the needs and risks of institutional closure programmes.

Larson F A, Larkin K C 1991 Parent attitude about residential placement before and after deinstitutionalisation. Journal of the Association for Persons with Severe Handicaps 16: 25–37

This is a research synthesis which offers the parental view of the policy decisions regarding reallocation programmes.

Reiter S 1991 Institutional reform – pre-requisites for providing a life of quality for mentally retarded residents. Research in Development Disabilities 12: 25–40

An evidence-based description which offers yardsticks and criteria for coordinated revision of residential services.

REFERENCES

Allport G W 1937 Personality, a psychological interpretation. Holt, Rinehart and Winston, New York
Audit Commission 1986 Making a reality of community care. HMSO, London
Bennis W G, Beene K D, Chin R, Carey K E 1976 The planning of change, 3rd edn. Holt, Rinehart and Winston, New York
Bulmer M 1987 The social basis of community care. Allen and Unwin, London
Davis-Jones H 1992 Social pedagogy: a description. In: Thompson T, Matthias P (eds) Standards and mental handicap-keys to competence. Baillière-Tindall, London
Farmer R, Rolde J, Sacks P 1991 Dimensions of mental handicap. Charing Cross and Westminster Medical School, London
Glynn J, Perkins D (eds) 1995 Managing health care – challenges for the 1990s. W B Saunders, London
Goodwin S 1989 Community care for the mentally ill in England and Wales; myths, assumptions and reality. Journal of Social Policy 18 (1): 27–52
Griffiths R 1988 Community care: agenda for action. HMSO, London
Ovretveit J, Mathias P, Thompson T (eds) 1997 Interprofessional working for health and social care. Macmillan, Basingstoke
Roos P, McCann B, Addison M 1980 Shaping the future. Community based residential services and facilities for mentally retarded people. University Park Press, Baltimore
Toffler A 1970 Future shock. Random House, New York
Twigg J, Atkin K 1994 Carers perceived: policy and practice in informal care. Open University Press, Buckingham
United Kingdom Central Council for Nursing, Midwifery and Health Visiting 1992 Code of conduct. UKCC, London
Wistow G 1985 Community care for the mentally handicapped: disappointing progress. In: Harrison A, Gretton J (eds) Health care UK. Policy Journals, London
Wolfensberger W 1972 Principles of normalisation in human services. National Institute of Mental Retardation, Toronto

Section 3

Evaluating changes to preparation

9. Mapping changing competences in the community adult nursing arena   *171*

10. Evidence-based nursing, evaluation and the role of the community practitioner   *197*

Mapping changing competences in the community adult nursing arena

Annette Lankshear   Carl Thompson

KEY ISSUES

- Policy change.
- Cultural separation and development of community nursing as a specialty.
- Research suggests that the work of community nurses is fundamentally different from that of other branches of nursing.
- The changing nature of illness and community-based clinical challenges.

INTRODUCTION

The conceptual links between competence and evaluation: outlining competence

There are a number of ways of making sense of the idea of competence in relation to work and employment. Something which almost all models of competence stress is an emphasis on either the inputs individuals make to work (such as aptitude, skills and knowledge) or, alternatively, the outcomes of work roles.

An input-based approach to competence might describe the everyday activity of patient assessment of pressure areas risk as: 'applies Waterlow scale' (this is a description of a task and yet also implies skills not specified such as assessment, degree of numeracy, risk management, etc.). An outcomes-based approach to the same task might express it as: 'produces personalized assessment of pressure area risk using Waterlow scale' (the outcome of the activity).

The dominant modes of thought in relation to competence can be summarized as a model (Fig. 9.1).

During the qualitative phase of the study it was apparent that the 'doing' part of the occupational role of being a nurse was as and in some cases more important than the endproduct or outcome of nursing per se. With this in mind and in the best traditions of discursive theory, we brought the two groups of models together so that the project took as its starting point the view that competence entails:

> ... *the ability to perform to an agreed standard, a specified set of tasks,*
> *processes and functions over an agreed range of contexts and situations.*
> (Eraut & Cole 1993)

Clearly, then, the task for the research team, in relation to the mapping of competences, was to identify those tasks, processes and functions and to do so in a way which was sensitive to the varied range of contexts and situations in which nurses operate.

From this definition the evaluatory agenda can be quickly gleaned as it relates to the issue of standards in occupations. The *raison d'être* of competence development is that elements of it can be made tangible and amenable to measurement and therefore can be evaluated. Our challenge was to find those elements which were most closely associated with the nursing role in institutional and community settings. No easy task, given that almost all the variables in the equation are relative in nature. What counts as occupational knowledge, skill, quality and performance can all be shown to have varying degrees of relativity attached.

We shall return to the issue of an agenda for evaluation later but for now the aim is simply to flag that, given the relative, shifting nature of the variables involved, we decided early on in the project that any methodology devised would have to be sufficiently sensitive to pick up on issues at the peripheries of these shifts and not to lose track of the fact that nurse education is in the business of turning out practitioners who are ready to practise competently. The aim of the study was to inform policy makers as to the environments most likely to:

> ... *secure sufficient clinical experience and supervision for students in*
> *practice placements to achieve specified learning outcomes and professional*
> *competencies.* (NHS Executive 1995: p. 6)

Expressed alternatively, the aim was a competence-based evaluation of community and institutional settings in relation to pre- and postregistration education and training needs.

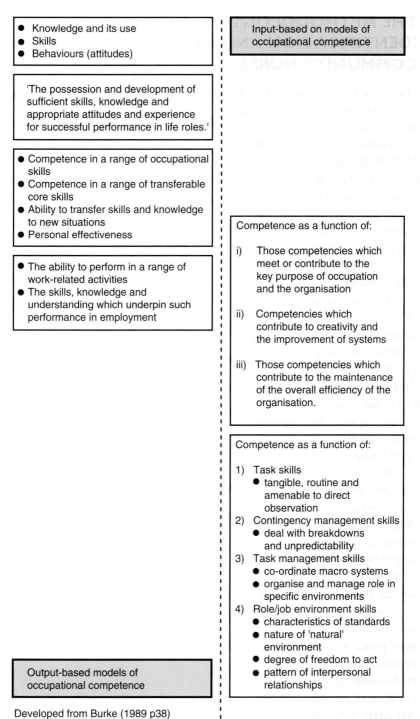

- Knowledge and its use
- Skills
- Behaviours (attitudes)

Input-based on models of occupational competence

'The possession and development of sufficient skills, knowledge and appropriate attitudes and experience for successful performance in life roles.'

- Competence in a range of occupational skills
- Competence in a range of transferable core skills
- Ability to transfer skills and knowledge to new situations
- Personal effectiveness

Competence as a function of:

i) Those competencies which meet or contribute to the key purpose of occupation and the organisation

- The ability to perform in a range of work-related activities
- The skills, knowledge and understanding which underpin such performance in employment

ii) Competencies which contribute to creativity and the improvement of systems

iii) Those competencies which contribute to the maintenance of the overall efficiency of the organisation.

Competence as a function of:

1) Task skills
   - tangible, routine and amenable to direct observation
2) Contingency management skills
   - deal with breakdowns and unpredictability
3) Task management skills
   - co-ordinate macro systems
   - organise and manage role in specific environments
4) Role/job environment skills
   - characteristics of standards
   - nature of 'natural' environment
   - degree of freedom to act
   - pattern of interpersonal relationships

Output-based models of occupational competence

Developed from Burke (1989 p38)

Fig. 9.1 Models of competence.

THE METHODOLOGY OF COMPETENCE IDENTIFICATION AND EXAMINATION IN COMMUNITY NURSES

The community nursing environment is a complex one; a plethora of variables can and do impact on the health profiles of the people who use community nursing services. Community nurses have little or no control over the environment in which they deliver care, unlike hospital-based nurses. Multiple disciplines, some of whom will lie outside the immediate multidisciplinary team (such as chiropodists), may be involved in an individual's health care. Transportation, community facilities, family or carer support and even the weather (community nurses in rural areas may not be able to reach patients) have a much greater impact on the roles and functions attached to community nursing. The task for a researcher seeking to establish a 'core' of the most rapidly changing areas of nursing competence in the community is to account for these confounding factors.

On a less contextual note, there are good methodological reasons why simply asking professionals, or groups aspiring to full 'professional' status, to define what makes them special or 'different' is not appropriate. A number of theorists have argued that one basis for professional power is the way in which, by simultaneously meeting patients' needs, they manage to legitimize their role and knowledge and therefore further their own professional interests at the same time (Williamson 1992). Moreover, once well established, the power of professional groups extends to being able to self-determine that which counts as 'need' in patients and even the knowledge base of interventions designed to meet these needs.

Other commentators point to the fact that professional groups who work in the same arena of practice also seek to assert their distinctive contributions and to secure and enhance their role and, by implication, their power base (Walby & Greenwell 1994). An example of this can be found in the claims of nurses to a special knowledge base (based on ideas of caring rather than simple treatment).

It follows, then, that by asking community nurses (regardless of whether one counts them as professionals or aspiring professionals) to define what makes their role in services (and therefore their contribution to health) 'special' then one risks simply mapping those perceptions which will act to most enhance their power within services rather than any objectively derived differences between their role and their hospital-based counterparts or indeed other professional groups. Given this problem, it seems logical to approach the question of identification and examination of competence from more than one angle. One means of doing this in a rigorous way is via the process of 'triangulation'.

The notion of triangulation has practical uses in the field of navigation. When you wish to locate your position when navigating you take bearings and fix-lines from two or more landmarks and then take the point at which the lines cross as your starting point. The same analogy can be applied to the question of identifying and examining competencies. In this case the bearings we took were from the landmarks of previously published literature, survey, qualitative interview and focus groups. We were fixing our conceptual position by establishing our locus between methods. By examining the notion of competence from four separate directions, it was assumed that the points at which their findings crossed would be reasonably trustworthy (an essential prerequisite for any research).

However, Hammersley & Atkinson point out that:

> *The aggregation of data from different sources will [not] unproblematically add up to a more complete picture.* (Hammersley & Atkinson 1983: p. 199)

Nevertheless, triangulation, even with the contradictions and complexities it often generates, gives the researcher the chance to theorize about a more complete picture than if one source of data is used alone. An explanation (theory) which can account for anomalies (or negative cases) is a much more robust theory than one derived from an approach less likely to generate such negative cases.

The aim of triangulation is simple and its advantages were described well by Walker:

> *Triangulation can add qualification to research that would otherwise be accepted uncritically ... and [methods] can also complement each other when the survey provides a context for the qualitative work which in turn permits commentary on the survey findings.* (Walker 1985: p. 16)

Research purists or those adherents to single methodological approaches may question the mixing of the qualitative and the quantitative paradigms in this study. One might argue, however, as Davies does, that the two are not as distinct as is sometimes proposed:

> *... methods* qua *techniques do not belong monopolistically to anyone. At root, what researchers do is extraordinarily simple: we look, ask and read. The organized form of these activities which we encounter within 'methods' books ... should not cause us to forget that observation, interviews, questionnaires ... are neither inherently qualitative or quantitative. All quantification involves judgement as to qualities and all qualitative statements invoke hierarchy, number and amount to give shape to meaning.* (Davies 1985: p. 290)

ESTABLISHING WAYMARKS – THE METHODS USED

Several data collection strategies were used in the study, each selected because of its appropriateness to researching the issue of 'competence' in institutional and community arenas.

The review of the literature

The literature review helped establish the conceptual framework for the study as well as outlining the professional, educational and governmental policy contexts within which the findings would have to be analysed. It set starting points for the gathering of empirical material by directly informing the interview schedules used in the qualitative work.

Semistructured interviews

Semistructured interviews took place with key players such as managers, GPs and nurses in the study. The semistructured interview was seen as combining the strengths of the unstructured interview (allowing for the immediate follow-up of pertinent issues raised by respondents) with the enhanced comparability between respondents of the structured interview. Every effort was made to allow respondents the chance to develop and voice ideas which diverted from the immediate topic guide and interview schedule where necessary.

The focus group

Nursing takes place in the context of alliances (for example, between nurses and patients, nurses and doctors, nurses and other nurses). Given this context, the focus group seemed a logical starting point for gathering material. The focus group has at its core a rationale stating that individuals neither form nor hold opinions in isolation. The technique of the focus group whereby a series of prompts are used as mechanisms for group-led discussion provides an excellent means of minimizing the researcher-led bias that can be a feature of semistructured interviews. Of course, the downside of this is that if groups are constructed badly then the views of one or two key individuals can dominate the discussion. This is a particular problem in health care where doctors and health care providers are discussing common issues within the same groups. The power dynamic that exists between the two groups in the workplace can be replicated within the focus group environment. The membership of these groups was broad enough to try and combat this. Participants included representatives from medicine, dietetics, social work, nursing, physiotherapy and psychology, amongst others.

Both of these qualitative approaches were aimed at understanding on the 'experience' of work. The perceptions of new challenges to old elements of competence. They dealt with the world of nursing from the viewpoint of the nurses, managers and doctors interviewed. They allowed us to develop conceptual categories for theorizing about competence and challenges within nursing. These methods, however, did not enable us to quantify these challenges, or allow us to weight the different elements of a nurse's role and to generalize to those nurses not immediately involved in the study – the technique used for this was the survey.

The survey

As already stated, the aim of the survey was to allow generalization about people rather than concepts. This was not as easy as it sounds, however. If surveys are to possess anything at all in the way of internal validity then they need a firm and established knowledge base on which to build. Competence is, conceptually speaking, still in its infancy; empirical analysis to help inform the development of knowledge is relatively rare and well-validated research findings scarce. Our problem, then, was twofold: namely, how could we maximize the internal validity of the survey instrument and at the same time remain 'sympathetic' to the largely qualitative paradigm within which the research was located? We addressed this by rigorous analysis of the qualitative material and using some of the conceptual categories developed from this as a means of 'framing' the subgroups used in the questionnaire. In this sense the items used could be considered 'grounded' in as much as they were derived from an analysis of the social world which was sensitive to change, adaptation and reflection. The survey sample was randomly selected from grade D–H nurse populations in three geographical areas. In all three institutional settings, this was by the use of staff lists and tables of random numbers. In the community settings it was carried out via a computerized random selection from computer data yielded from the local FHSA staff lists. A total of 630 questionnaires were sent out (585 adult and mental health nurses and 45 practice nurses) and 419 were returned, giving a total response rate of approximately 67%.

WHAT DID WE FIND?

There were a number of 'themes' which ran through both the qualitative and quantitative data.

◆ A sense of difference between the skills and roles involved in community nursing versus those required in hospital was evident in nurses' responses.
◆ Probably because of this, opportunities for developing some competences were almost 'exclusive' to community or hospital settings.

◆ The introduction of large-scale social policies such as the community care component of the NHS and Community Care Act was influencing new nursing roles and associated competences.

The survey asked nurses to rate how often an observer could expect to see them carrying out any of the competences developed from the qualitative component of the study and also how important they felt the competence element was to their future role. The competences were grouped together under logical categories such as 'clinical evaluation' which enabled us to transform the ordinal data into a non-categorical 'average' for each group of competences.

The original ordinal data for each element of competence was analysed for differences between hospital, community and combined settings using the Kruskall-Wallis non-parametric analysis of variance (corrected for ties). Differences in the 'scores' for each group of competences were analysed using independent t-tests using the settings (hospital or community) as the grouping variables.

This analysis allowed us to examine the differences in importance and frequency for each competence according to hospital and community settings but also to recommend placement areas where elements of competence might best be gained.

Table 9.1 outlines those differences between hospital and community settings in relation to how regularly an observer might expect to see the competence as part of the nurse's role.

Table 9.2 presents the same groups of competences but this time in relation to how important nurses feel they are to their future role.

Table 9.3 breaks down some of these grouped competencies and presents those individual elements of competence which are best observed in either hospital or community settings.

HORSES FOR COURSES – DIFFERENT CARE SETTINGS, DIFFERENT SKILLS AND COMPETENCES?

What these figures represent is a somewhat delineated picture of the different skills and competences involved in nursing in community and institutional settings. Of the 13 groups of competences identified from the qualitative work, over half were seen to have significant differences in the frequency with which they might be observed in practice. Six of these were most closely associated with nursing in community settings:

◆ context of care
◆ patient-centred care

◆ nursing actions
◆ clinical evaluation
◆ personal and professional development
◆ managing change

whilst the issue of nursing skills development appeared to favour the hospital environment.

In terms of perceived importance to nurses in their future role, the picture was less segmented. The issues of context of care and nursing actions were more positively valued by community nurses, whilst the grouped

Table 9.1 The groups of competences observed (scale of 1–5). Lowest score = most regularly observed

Area of competence	Setting	Mean
Context of care*	Community	1.65
	Hospital	2.32
Patient-centred care*	Community	1.8
	Hospital	1.9
Clinical assessment	Community	1.9
	Hospital	1.8
Nursing actions**	Community	2.2
	Hospital	2.5
Nursing skills**	Community	2.8
	Hospital	2.5
Clinical evaluation**	Community	2.1
	Hospital	2.4
Multidisciplinary working	Community	2.2
	Hospital	2.1
Research	Community	2.3
	Hospital	2.2
Personal and professional development*	Community	1.9
	Hospital	2.1
Education	Community	1.9
	Hospital	1.9
Managing change**	Community	2.4
	Hospital	2.6
Management	Community	2.1
	Hospital	2.1
Communication	Community	1.6
	Hospital	1.7

Community n = 115
Hospital n = 95
 * p>.05
** p>.01

Table 9.2 The groups of competences: importance (scale of 1–5). High score = most important

Area of competence	Setting	Mean
Context of care**	Community	2.7
	Hospital	2.2
Patient-centred care	Community	2.6
	Hospital	2.6
Clinical assessment	Community	2.6
	Hospital	2.6
Nursing actions**	Community	2.4
	Hospital	2.2
Nursing skills**	Community	1.8
	Hospital	2.3
Clinical evaluation	Community	2.6
	Hospital	2.5
Multidisciplinary working	Community	2.5
	Hospital	2.6
Research	Community	2.7
	Hospital	2.8
Personal and professional development	Community	2.8
	Hospital	2.8
Education*	Community	2.6
	Hospital	2.7
Managing change	Community	2.5
	Hospital	2.4
Management	Community	2.5
	Hospital	2.5
Communication	Community	2.9
	Hospital	2.9

Community n = 115
Hospital n = 95
 $* p > .05$
$** p > .01$

competences of nursing skills and education found favour with their hospital-based counterparts.

Appendix A shows the constituent parts of each competence group, giving the reader a 'flavour' of the significance for evaluating practice of the differences highlighted by the survey.

One of the problems of a quantitative exercise such as this is that on their own, the findings only highlight a small part of the dilemma facing the educationalist who seeks to prepare nurses by placing them in situations which will allow their skills to be evaluated in 'real-life' scenarios and in which preparation will have a large experiential component, with the relevant mentorship

Table 9.3 The best settings in which to observe specific competences

Community settings	Hospital settings
◆ Having patient contact in both hospital and community settings	◆ Participating in decisions related to resuscitation based on quality of life indicators
◆ Undertaking practice sensitive to the needs of patients from multicultural backgrounds	◆ Assessing neurological function
◆ Working in conjunction with the voluntary and private sectors	◆ Making a daily assessment of all clients for whom I am responsible
◆ Negotiating and retaining access to patients' homes	◆ Recognizing the effects of prescribed drugs and drug interactions
◆ Undertaking nursing practice in settings physically remote from colleagues	◆ Carrying out physical assessment of clients
◆ Dealing with issues related to public health	◆ Adjusting patient medication in response to laboratory findings
◆ Undertaking health-screening programmes	◆ Carrying out intubation/extubation
◆ Fostering autonomy in relation to health-care decisions	◆ Managing and monitoring CVP lines
◆ Maintaining and monitoring long-term relationships with individuals, families or other social groups for health maintenance	◆ Taking blood from arterial lines
	◆ Carrying out defibrillation
◆ Undertaking comprehensive health-care needs assessment of communities	◆ Inserting a peripheral cannula
	◆ Administration of IV drugs
◆ Making and acting upon decisions which carry risks to families	◆ Assisting with the induction of anaesthesia
◆ Making and acting upon decisions which carry risks to communities	◆ Assisting the surgeon
	◆ Assisting with tracheostomy formation
◆ Transporting drugs outside hospital premises	◆ Interpreting X-rays
◆ Administration and disposing of medicines outside the hospital situation	◆ Actively working with consultants
	◆ Actively working with pharmacists
◆ Interpreting and applying the Community Care Act	◆ Coordinating the multidisciplinary team in discharge planning
◆ Interpreting and applying the Children Act	◆ Collaborating with the multidisciplinary team in reaching decisions in ethically challenging situations
◆ Attending court hearings/tribunals and engagement with the criminal justice system	
◆ Attending child protection meetings	◆ Actively working with physiotherapists
◆ Allocating patients to diagnostic groups on the basis of treatment initiated	◆ Actively working with ODAs
◆ Facilitating group therapy meetings	◆ Identifying researchable problems
◆ Running cervical cytology clinics	◆ Operating as a mentor for students and staff
◆ Carrying out male catheterization	◆ Assessing NVQ competencies
◆ Undertaking breast examination	◆ Participating in clinical supervision
◆ Using computer-held data to inform client care outcomes evaluation	◆ Disseminating information about education resources and opportunities
◆ Undertaking evaluation strategies with the aid of audit tools	

contd

Table 9.3 (contd)

Community settings	Hospital settings
◆ Accessing local databases held on computer	◆ Supporting junior medical colleagues
◆ Accessing national databases on computer	◆ Monitoring the actions of others to whom patient care has been delegated
◆ Actively participating in multidisciplinary meetings	
◆ Actively working with chiropodists/ podiatrists	◆ Managing the allocation of patients to a multiskilled team
◆ Actively working with GPs	◆ Managing a budget
◆ Participating in meetings in which decisions are made regarding the selection of key workers	◆ Writing discharge letters to GPs
	◆ Dealing personally with patients/ families/carers who make a complaint
◆ Actively working with audiologists	
◆ Identifying researchable problems	
◆ Completing reflective diaries	
◆ Undertaking informal health education activities with families or carers	
◆ Delivering formal health-education activities to individuals	
◆ Delivering formal health-education activities to families	
◆ Educating patients/carers in the use of equipment in community settings	
◆ Contributing to meetings at which broad professional issues are discussed	
◆ Reviewing workload priorities as a response to changing contexts	
◆ Inputting data to computerized management information systems	
◆ Managing nurse-led clinics	
◆ Initiating and maintaining the use of client-held records	
◆ Using counselling skills in dealings with clients	

models a realistic proposition. Any evaluation of training settings has to include more than simply the 'quantity' of training opportunities; it has also to encompass the 'quality' of those settings.

One way of easing this dilemma and aiding assessments of the appropriateness, fitness for purpose or 'quality' of the settings is to take a qualitative perspective in order to add depth and richness to a quantitative 'map' of the competences in place. The principle can be demonstrated with reference to two of the areas in which delineation between types of work and associated competences were most in evidence in this study: the areas affected by the 'context of care' and those issues encompassed within the category of 'nursing skills'.

Context of care

The drive to centre care in the patient's home whenever possible had had the effect that traditional boundaries between hospital and community care were gradually becoming less clear. Early signs of such boundary changes are described by a nurse manager in medical services.

> *We have a dermatology nurse specialist who sees them on the ward, sees them on the outpatients and outside into the community. We used to have in situ 20 odd dermatology beds, now we've got 12 going down to about 10, but there's more resources going into the outpatients for somebody to be seeing them, so gone are the days now nursing people over weeks really, rather days, and so therefore what facilities are required after discharge or even before discharge or before admission really, it's more concentration on that.*

One trust in the study had elected to develop an outreach facility for its major elective orthopaedic surgery. The remit of the outreach nurse was to achieve a shortening of the length of stay, which he had done by establishing pre-assessment clinics, visiting patients on the ward to give further information about their surgery and convalescence and then following them up at home after early discharge. If they needed any sort of intervention, he would respond until the 14th postoperative day, in the words of one respondent, 'similar to a midwife'. It would appear that the specific clinical expertise of the specialist nurse was valued by the medical staff and offered a safeguard to both senior nursing and medical teams in the management of risk inherent in the implementation of these new initiatives. The specialist expertise thus made available was deemed to be worth the inefficiency of one nurse visiting patients over a wide geographical area. Consultant medical staff were simply not confident that district nurses were equipped to offer contemporary research-based orthopaedic nursing care. However, a senior director of community services took the view that another skill set was being devalued.

> *I have discussed with many hospital nurses in the past their ability to move away from the hospital setting and into somebody's home. (They) think they can do that relatively easily … they feel that nursing on the ward is exactly the same as nursing in somebody's home, which is a very naive view.*

The following extracts, from practitioners with recent experience in carrying out home visits for the first time, bear out this viewpoint.

Well, you are going to the client as opposed to them coming to you, and knocking on doors is horrid at first.

You are on their territory, if they don't wish to see you, they will close the door. You need to improve your communication skills – what you need to do if you are in a situation where you have a very aggressive client and you're on your own ... where do you sit, how do you diffuse aggression.

Within the hospital setting it can be relatively easy to defer decisions and to refer issues to other more senior practitioners. Indeed, many aspects of the hierarchy and organizational structure promote this behaviour. Respondents who work in community settings emphasized the isolated nature of their working patterns and, from time to time, the need to make decisions without discussion with medical and nursing colleagues. They highlighted the accompanying stress which this brings.

You are on your own, you have to make decisions and you have to be held accountable for that and that feels very different. (District nurse)

Especially when you've now got the situation that you've got here that you're totally isolated really, aren't you. You're not anywhere near the GPs. (Outreach nurse)

At ward level it wasn't too bad, you did have other colleagues around you when things were going up the creek but I think in the community because of the isolation of the job you couldn't forget where you are and end up with stress without even recognizing the symptoms. (Outreach nurse)

Decision making is often based on experience, but with new situations being faced with more acute patients being nursed in the community, experience may have to give way to untried solutions which must be constantly evaluated.

One outcome of the increase in community care was the rising importance of the provision made within the independent sector. Given the demographic changes occurring concomitantly with bed reductions, reliance on the continued development of provision by the independent and voluntary sectors was high. There were expectations that the range of services offered outside the NHS would continue to grow; relationships with charitable organizations were also discussed. In one area the charity Age Concern was providing a service to elderly patients attending A & E, with volunteers accompanying elderly attendees and taking care of domestic problems such as abandoned pets. Trust dependence on the fundraising activities of charities was also acknowledged, as was the group home provision of such bodies as the Schizophrenia Fellowship and the educational role of the British Diabetic Society and the Heart Foundation.

Specific nursing skills

The reduction in the hours worked by junior hospital doctors heralded by the publication of 'A New Deal' (Department of Health 1991) had facilitated a review of many areas of work traditionally undertaken by this group. This, combined with the publication of the UKCC's 'The Scope of Professional Practice' (UKCC 1992) had led to a redefinition of the boundary between medicine and nursing. The report of the Audit Commission on the work of hospital doctors in England and Wales stated that:

> ... *hospitals differ in how tasks are divided between junior doctors and nurses and other professional groups. In many hospitals nurses and other professionals are now working in areas traditionally regarded as the province of doctors.* (Audit Commission 1995: p. 18)

In addition to specific skills and roles, new posts have been created. During the course of the study, we interviewed a 'bed manager' – a nurse manager whose role was developed to relieve junior doctors of the responsibility of finding beds for acute admissions.

Developments are taking place in A & E departments, with nurses taking responsibility for diagnosis and treatment of a range of injuries. Nurses are undertaking triage, ordering X-rays and assigning patients to doctors for advice or to nurses for treatment. Within defined protocols, nurses, particularly those in community hospitals, are diagnosing and treating fractures, treating minor burns and scalds, suturing and stapling wounds, administering antibiotics and tetanus toxoid within protocols, dispensing simple analgesics, removing foreign bodies and advising those with head injuries.

In September 1994, after the completion of the interview phase of the study, the Greenhalgh Report was published. This identified a total of 79 enhanced/extended role activities identified from the 10 sites visited by the research team. The report argued that 75% of junior hospital doctor time was spent on just seven activities:

- ◆ insertion of a peripheral IV cannula;
- ◆ venous blood sampling;
- ◆ administration of drugs (excluding cytotoxic and first dose) via a peripheral IV cannula;
- ◆ urethral catheterization of male patients;
- ◆ taking patient histories;
- ◆ referring patients for investigations;
- ◆ writing and signing discharge letters (Greenhalgh & Co 1994).

While all these activities were cited by respondents in this study as forming part of the role of the nurse in the future, four in particular were especially prominent: insertion of a peripheral IV cannula, venous blood sampling, administration of drugs (excluding cytotoxic and first dose) via a peripheral IV cannula and urethral catheterization of male and female patients. A fifth skill also mentioned by several of the respondents in this study, although not on the list above, was the recording of 12-lead ECGs. Senior managers were adamant that all practitioners should have these skills within their repertoire in order to demonstrate fitness for purpose and that they should feature in the outcomes of preregistration education for Part 12 of the register. Whilst the immediate impetus for change came from the need to introduce the recommendations of 'The New Deal', there was as previously stated an explicit recognition that the changes provided an opportunity to increase the efficiency and acceptability of the service provided to patients.

> *At the moment the night sisters from both hospitals are in the planning stages of developing a night practitioner's role which the director of nursing services is involved in, setting up the training scheme for us to go to, and to extend our role into a different job altogether really. They are wanting us to do limited prescribing, learn catheterization, ECGs, obviously intravenous drugs and venepuncture and verifying expected deaths.* (Manager)

Practitioners speaking in the focus groups agreed that the extension to their role provided patients with appropriate treatments at appropriate times and generally enhanced the smooth running of the ward environment.

> *Well, we have now started to give intravenous drugs … well, it is a good idea because sometimes when you are trying to get hold of a doctor and they are busy in theatre or with an emergency, etc. the patient tends not to get the intravenous drugs on time such as antibiotics so then you've got a domino effect where they are always behind so you have to give the next dose later on, etc., etc. We are also starting to do venepuncture as well, we have been doing study days on that as well and also ECGs as well.* (Practitioner)

Some respondents identified the development, in their own practice, of having a waiting list; formerly referrals would have been picked up by other members of the nursing team. As specialist nurses they plan and prioritize care, have their own referral system and may have their own budget. However, the practitioners felt that they had been inadequately consulted about the changes to their practice.

> *Nobody has actually asked nurses what they mind taking on but you are told, you know, you are going to have to do the cannulas.* (Practitioner)

> *Also they want us to venesect patients and put drips up and they are looking at reducing the working day of the doctor so that is bound to mean more jobs going to the nurse because that is what the nurses are for. The nurses*

will do it, how many times have we all heard that, 'Oh, the nurses will do it'.
(Practitioner)

Further evidence of the changing role lies in the claim that nurses are admitting and discharging patients within defined protocols. The following statements were made by senior managers in different trusts.

Extending more in nursing assessment, perhaps we did a few years ago and the scope of practice has allowed us to do that. For example, on coronary care we admit people. You know a GP will ring, a nurse will say right, he's got a chest pain, he's got an ECG of this and he must come into coronary care.

Nurses are now looking ... to advise on discharge ... traditionally it's always been the doctor that's done it. So that's changing now. Five day ward – the nurses discharge the patients, because if they wait for the doctor it would be chaos. By the time they got there there'd be too many patients and not enough beds ... they have a set criteria which is discussed between the nurse and the doctor.

There is, however, another side to this coin. For adult nurses the notion of professional accountability is in the forefront, linked with the need to be assertive. On occasion, nurses would refuse to admit patients when there were no available beds. At the other end of the patient episode, they refused to send patients home inappropriately and refused to put up extra beds on the ward. 'Professional accountability', said one senior manager, 'requires assertion skills. Life is a constant juggling act.'

As the impact of the NHS and Community Care Act is felt not only are patients discharged early from hospitals but patients who may have traditionally been admitted to hospital are being looked after at home.

I had a lady recently, she's in hospital now but has endstage cor pulmonale ... woman who's getting totally breathless just walking to the toilet and back yet was at home rather than being admitted to hospital because, OK, there's nothing particular. I mean, they can give her some drugs but ... there's nothing life saving probably they can do. So more people I would say are staying at home. (District nurse)

Respondents suggested that as nurses in the community are increasingly charged with the continuity of care in complex care scenarios, such as stroke rehabilitation, it is evident that the skills required are becoming more complex. Many respondents made reference to the highly technical nature of care with which district nurses will have to deal. Skills required range from the intravenous administration of cytotoxic drugs to management of patient-controlled systems of analgesia, parenteral feeding systems and so forth. One

GP respondent expressed his views on the future of community nursing and the potential implications for his work arising from the increasingly technical nature of client care in the community.

> *I think nurses do a lot of the terminal care and pain control that was always done in hospital. I think in the future you're going to get intravenous feeding ... care of cystic fibrosis children with IV lines to maintain, IV antibiotics, care of neonates more in the community. You're going to get care of adult patients needing regular IVs, chronic chests and the like, bronchitis patients.*

Also in keeping with this, district nurses reported that they were providing home care to patients with complex technical equipment or supporting and administering intravenous therapy to patients in their own homes.

> *We're looking into IV training and Hickman line training because people ... coming home, they're on chemotherapy ... and we've looked at what impact that's having on the service and the one thing we can see in the very near future, because we're already getting them home. In other areas of the country there are actually district nurses giving IVs to patients at home.*
> (Middle manager)

In recognition of this increasing trend, the ENB published the final report of the working group on 'Developing the Role of the District Nurse in the Administration of Intravenous Therapy in the Home' (ENB 1994). It recognized that DNs were being increasingly required to manage Hickman lines and portacaths for clients requiring long-term therapy (such as those with HIV and AIDS). One year later, the publication of the NHSE letter EL(95/5) 'Purchasing High Tech Health Care for Patients at Home' recognized the implications of funding packages of care such as CAPD and total parenteral nutrition and decreed that these should be part of the formal contract between purchasers and providers.

Multidisciplinary working

In the acute trusts, a wide range of professionals joined the groups to discuss the concept of teamworking. It was evident from the discussion that the range of experiences of interprofessional working was broad, varying from excellent to non-existent. Examples of good practice were cited in specialty areas such as care of the elderly, rheumatology and neurology. In the area of general medicine and surgery, however, the respondents reported that there were no meetings of a multidisciplinary nature and that there was a general lack of understanding of the roles of various professionals involved in the care and treatment of patients.

> *I don't think there's many people round this table actually knows what the person next to them does.* (Senior house officer)

I think even in a hospital that … that you still get … the confusion and … you still get teams that don't actually work necessarily together on a daily basis. (Speech and language therapist)

Apart from the well-defined areas of good practice mentioned, the picture emerged of a multitude of professionals entering a ward (where they may not even be known), carrying out an assessment, making therapeutic interventions, reporting the outcome to the nursing staff and leaving. There was no occasion for all concerned with the care of patients to sit down together and attempt to piece together a complete picture. Whilst no-one believed this lack of formal communication to be in the patient's best interest, it was believed that such was the pace of life on busy medical and surgical wards that sitting down to discuss a patient was a luxury that no-one could afford. The multidisciplinary team (MDT) respondents typically covered several wards and were under pressure to treat all the inpatients referred to them. One expressed a feeling of being trapped into traditional patterns of behaviour by traditional patterns of funding. He could not envisage, in the present climate of performance indicators, being able to successfully argue a case in which he treated fewer patients to a higher quality.

Several respondents from both acute and mental health services commented that it was still the norm for the leadership of team, where it meets regularly, to rest with the consultant who chairs it and directs its business. This despite the view of Spratley & Pietroni (1994) who claim that doctors are trained and socialized into a system that requires them to make difficult decisions autonomously and without consultation with others – a perspective antithetical to that of the multidisciplinary team. A middle manager in forensic services offered an explanation for this phenomenon.

Probably because a lot of years ago they were called doctors' ward rounds and even though the title's changed to clinical review meetings or something like that, it's just continued … the multidisciplinary team meeting is a direct descendant of the ward round.

Senior house officers in an acute trust remarked:

It depends on the consultant very much. I mean, a lot of the younger ones … are much more … willing to involve with the people in the management of their patients.

I think … a lot of it's due to the attitude of … the medical staff as well. Even though they're not supposed to be the centre of it, if they insist on having it and … sit and listen to people then it's more likely to continue on and people get a better deal.

Everything has to go by the psychiatrist really and then he will direct the work, so it's patchy.

Whilst nurses were certainly not seen as natural leaders of the MDT, the view expressed consistently by nurses and their managers that they occupied a central position in the multidisciplinary team was strongly upheld by hospital-based members of the MDT in both acute and mental health settings.

> *It tends to be the nursing staff who are central to the multidisciplinary team because they are there in the inpatient setting, they are there ... 24 hours a day, whereas the rest of us might drift in and out.* (Physiotherapist)

> *I think the doctors like to think that ... they're the coordinators, but in fact it's usually the nursing sisters and the staff nurses.* (Senior house officer)

> *We perhaps depend on a nurse to give us clear information about what another member of the, quotes, team is doing.* (Social worker)

> *I certainly think the nurse is the link between everybody else and the team, because they're the ones who are there with the patient all the time.* (Dietitian)

> *If you were to remove the nurse the patient just wouldn't carry on, do you know what I mean. I can't see how the patient could be cared for by all the little bits.* (Senior nurse manger)

> *I think sometimes on a ward the nurse plays that central, sort of, coordinating role, it's not a lead role, but it's just ... you know, has everybody been in contact with everybody.* (Senior house officer)

In contrast, care in the community for the physically sick is seen as a fragmented activity, with a large number of professionals visiting patients, frequently unaware of how many others are also engaged in treatment. The multidisciplinary team do not view the nurse as the obvious coordinator in this setting. With the loss of the 24-hour nursing presence (if not of the 24-hour responsibility) respondents reported that the patient assumes the central role as the only person who has an holistic view of the care being given.

> *For example, people with motor neurone disease and there can be 14 different people going into that person's house ... (all) part of a multidisciplinary team. The only person who knows everybody is the patient themselves.*

> *I think it's from social services though that it's coming in the community, that they're recognizing that there is usually a coordinator. But it isn't necessarily a nurse.*

CONCLUSION

This chapter has demonstrated that institutional and community settings offer fundamentally different learning experiences for the nursing student. The full report upon which the chapter was based details how these differ. But the primary usefulness of this chapter relates to how it demonstrates that mixed research methods can appropriately act as a framework for exploring the quantity and quality of learning opportunities and chances for competence development in both institutional and community settings. It has explored some of the most rapidly changing areas of the nurse's role, especially those which have arisen as part of broader shifts in the contexts of care within which nurses must operate. These contexts, which include a blurring of the boundary between acute secondary care and the primary arena, have tangible effects on the role expectations and importance nurses attach to elements of their skills portfolio.

In conclusion, we suggest that a competence-based approach to evaluating settings for learning opportunities has much to offer the educationalist seeking to contribute to the production of nurses who are fit for the purposes of nursing in the 21st century and the development of occupational standards which meet the needs not just of our profession and care environments, but of the public we serve.

QUESTIONS FOR DISCUSSION

◆ Are there alternative elements of a nurse's competence you might wish to examine if you were responsible for commissioning health services?

◆ How useful do you think the concept of competence is to a discussion of the value of nursing in health services?

◆ Does the notion of competence help or hinder nurses' efforts to be seen as more 'professional' in the health-care arena?

ANNOTATED BIBLIOGRAPHY

Tuxworth E 1992 Beyond the basics – higher level competence. In: Thompson T, Mathias P (eds) Standards and mental handicap: keys to competence. Baillière Tindall, London

This is an excellent introduction to the conceptual issues surrounding competence and its assessment. It manages to achieve the right blend of readability and depth of application.

Eraut M 1994 Developing professional knowledge and competence. Falmer Press, London

The author is Professor of Education at the University of Sussex and his broad range of publications are testimony to his wide-ranging, multiprofessional grasp of the concept of competence.

Burke J W (ed) (1989) Competency based education and training. Falmer Press, London

This is an essential read for anyone wishing to understand the core elements of a competence-based approach to professional preparation. The first five chapters in particular are especially useful to a discussion of nursing, with issues such as defining standards, the competence–knowledge 'mix' and the origins of competence all brought to the fore.

Lankshear A, Brown J, Thompson C 1996 Practice placement project: mapping the nursing competencies required in institutional and community settings in the context of multidisciplinary health care provision (an exploratory study). English National Board for Nursing, Midwifery and Health Visiting, London

This is the full report, upon which this chapter is based. It deals with 'hard' issues of where best to observe and develop competences in clinical settings as well as having significant chapters on the methodology of competence observation and its conceptual relevance to nursing.

REFERENCES

Audit Commission 1995 The doctor's tale: the work of hospital doctors in England and Wales. HMSO, London
Davies B 1985 Integrating methodologies. In: Burgess R G (ed) Strategies of educational research. Falmer Press, London
Department of Health 1991 Doctors in training: a new deal. HMSO, London
English National Board 1994 Developing the role of the district nurse in the administration of intra-venous therapy in the home. ENB, London
Eraut M 1994 Developing professional knowledge and competence. Falmer Press, London
Greenalgh & Company Ltd 1994 The interface between junior doctors and nurses: a research study for the Department of Health. DoH, London
Hammersley M, Atkinson P 1983 Ethnography: principles and practice. Routledge, London
NHS Executive 1995 Education and training in the new NHS. EL95:27. NHS Executive, London
Salvage J 1992 The new nursing: empowering patients or empowering nurses? In: Robinson J et al (eds) Policy issues in nursing. Open University Press, Milton Keynes
United Kingdom Central Council 1992 The scope of professional practice. UKCC, London
Spratley J, Pietroni M 1994 Creative collaboration: inter-professional learning priorities in primary health and community care. Report of a project undertaken by the Marylebone Centre Trust on behalf of CCETSW, Marylebone Centre Trust, London
Walby S, Greenwell J 1994 Medicine and nursing: professions in a changing health service. Sage, London
Walker R L 1985 Applied qualitative research. Gower, Aldershot
Wiliamson C (1992) Whose standards: consumer and professional standards in health care. Open University Press, Buckingham

APPENDIX A CONSTITUENTS OF COMPETENCE GROUPS

Context of care

Having patient/client contact in both hospital and community settings

Undertaking practice sensitive to the needs of patients/clients from multi-cultural backgrounds
Working in conjunction with the voluntary and private sector
Negotiating and retaining access to patients'/clients' homes
Undertaking nursing practice in settings physically remote from colleagues
Dealing with issues related to public health
Undertaking health-screening programmes

Patient/client-centred care

Fostering autonomy of patients/clients in relation to health-care decisions
Maintaining and monitoring long-term relationships with individuals, families or other social groups for health maintenance
Making appropriate referrals when patients/clients seek legal advice
Acting as patient/client advocate regarding quality of life issues
Participating in decisions related to resuscitation based on quality of life indicators

Clinical assessment

Undertaking comprehensive health-care needs assessment of individuals
Undertaking comprehensive health-care needs assessment of families
Undertaking comprehensive health-care needs assessment of communities
Assessing social/life skills
Assessing neurological function
Taking the final decision to admit patients/clients to hospital within protocol criteria
Making a daily assessment of all clients for whom I am responsible
Recognizing the effects of prescribed drugs and drug interactions
Carrying out physical assessment of patients/clients

Nursing actions

Making and acting upon decisions which carry risks to patients/clients
Making and acting upon decisions which carry risks to families
Making and acting upon decisions which carry risks to communities
Making and acting upon decisions which carry risks to the organization
Transporting drugs outside hospital premises
Administering and disposing of medicines (including controlled drugs) outside the hospital situation
Interpreting and applying health and safety legislation
Interpreting and applying the Community Care Act
Interpreting and applying the Children Act
Interpreting and applying the Mental Health Act
Attending court hearings/tribunals and engagement with the criminal justice system

Attending meetings called for the purpose of child protection

Allocating patients/clients to diagnostic groups on the basis of which treatment is initiated

Facilitating group therapy meetings

Specific nursing skills

Adjusting patient medication in response to laboratory findings

Interpreting blood results and adjusting treatment accordingly

Confirming expected death

Prescribing drugs within protocols

Carrying out incubation and/or extubation

Managing and monitoring central venous pressure lines

Taking blood from arterial lines

Carrying out venepuncture

Carrying out defibrillation

Inserting a peripheral IV cannula

Initiating an IV regimen within protocols

Administration of IV drugs

Running cervical cytology clinics

Carrying out male catheterization

Assisting with the induction of anaesthesia

Assisting the surgeon

Assisting with tracheostomy formation in critical care environments

Removing foreign bodies from the eye

Interpreting X-rays

Undertaking breast examination

Undertaking pelvic or prostate examination

Clinical evaluation

Using computer-held data to inform the evaluation of client care outcomes

Undertaking evaluation strategies with the use of audit tools

Accessing local databases held on computer

Accessing national databases held on computer

Planning systems of nursing activity which satisfy agreed standards at local, unit or district level

Evaluating quality improvements to assure the ongoing quality of nursing services

Participating in multidisciplinary clinical audit

Multidisciplinary working

Actively participating in multidisciplinary team meetings

Actively working with social workers

Actively working with occupational therapists
Actively working with chiropodists/podiatrists
Actively working with dietitians
Actively working with consultants
Actively working with psychologists
Actively working with GPs
Actively working with pharmacists
Participating in meetings in which decisions are made regarding selection of key workers
Coordinating the multidisciplinary team in discharge planning
Participating in multidisciplinary standard setting
Participating in the writing of shared protocols for care
Collaborating with the multidisciplinary team in reaching clinical decisions in ethically challenging situations
Contributing to shared multidisciplinary team patient notes/records
Actively working with physiotherapists
Actively working with speech therapists
Actively working with audiologists
Actively working with operating department assistants (ODAs)

Research
Identifying researchable problems
Writing or collaborating in writing a research proposal
Communicating research findings to staff through formal and informal processes
Effecting change based on research findings
Critically analysing the findings of research studies

Personal and professional development
Completing reflective diaries
Maintaining a personal and professional portfolio

Education
Undertaking informal health-education activities with individuals
Undertaking informal health-education activities with families and carers
Operating as a mentor for students and staff
Assessing National Vocational Qualifications (NVQ) competences
Assessing student nurses
Participating in a process of clinical supervision
Disseminating information about educational resources and opportunities to staff

Delivering formal health-education activities/programmes to individuals
Delivering formal health-education activities/programmes to families
Supporting junior medical colleagues
Educating patients/clients/carers in the use of equipment in community settings

Managing change

Contributing to meetings regarding the business strategy of the trust
Contributing to meetings at which broad professional issues are discussed
Formally presenting a case for change

Management

Reviewing workload priorities as a response to changing contexts
Monitoring the actions of others to whom responsibility for patient/client care has been delegated
Managing the allocation of patients/clients to a multiskilled team
Managing care within the context of change
Dealing with formal requests for information from organizations outside the National Health Service
Chairing meetings
Inputting data to computerized information management systems
Managing a budget
Managing personnel issues and policies
Negotiating a care package for individual patients/clients
Taking the final decision to discharge patients/clients within defined protocols
Writing discharge letters to GPs
Managing nurse-led clinics
Initiating and maintaining the use of patient/client-held records

Communication

Using counselling skills in dealings with clients
Using counselling skills in dealings with their families
Using counselling skills in dealings with colleagues
Dealing personally with patients, their families or carers who make a complaint

Evidence-based nursing- evaluation and the role of the community practitioner

Jacqueline Droogan

KEY ISSUES

♦ Variations in clinical practice.

♦ Clinical effectiveness – doing more good than harm.

♦ The Information Systems Strategy (ISS).

♦ The research evidence.

♦ Dissemination.

♦ Nursing and the National Health Service Research and Development (NHS R&D) programme.

INTRODUCTION

This chapter explores some of the implications for community nurses of the shift within the NHS away from traditional modes of health-care delivery towards interventions based on the best available evidence – a shift towards evidence-based health care. The chapter dispels the myths surrounding evidence-based health care in relation to nursing, myths often upheld by nurses themselves. These myths include nurses not being able to undertake rigorous evaluative research and that research designs such as randomized controlled trials and systematic reviews cannot be applied to nursing care.

Variations in practice: the example of leg ulcers

Most district and practice nurses will have to deal with the treatment of leg ulcers at some time in their career. Preferences for particular types of dressings differ from team to team and from nurse to nurse. These differences represent wide-ranging variations in practice. Such variations are not just symptomatic of variations in nursing or the area of wound care, but also apply to other health care professions and interventions and in national and international contexts.

Variations in practice can occur because of differences in factors like population demographics, illness rates, the way local groups practise and the beliefs local professional groups hold about the effectiveness of differing techniques. For example, decisions about which dressing(s) to apply to a venous leg ulcer might be influenced by:

◆ an individual's belief about what has been found to work best, often based on reflections of personal clinical experience;
◆ discussion with professional colleagues and/or local experts such as the clinical nurse specialist;
◆ an article recommending a specific type of dressing;
◆ visits from pharmaceutical representatives promoting products;
◆ textbooks;
◆ nurse training and specialist continuing education programmes.

Most health care professionals strive to find the most effective intervention to treat a health care problem. However, the underlying sources of information which professionals draw on, and the contexts in which interventions are used, often vary.

Moreover, the same problem is not always treated in the same way by different health care professionals (Entwistle et al 1996). As a consequence, some patients will receive effective treatments whilst others receive treatments that are less effective and may do more harm than good.

Growing awareness of variations in practice throughout the whole of the health care arena raises questions about the role of scientific evidence in health care interventions. These questions form one of the triggers for a new approach to health care, namely, one which is evidence based (Entwistle et al 1996). There has been a move away from basing clinical decisions purely on tradition or expert opinion towards using the best available research evidence to help guide a particular decision or treatment. Other factors which have influenced the shift to evidence-based health care include:

◆ **population ageing:** people are living longer and the number of older people is increasing. This creates increasing age-related demand for health-care services. Such demands in turn create clinical and cost-related challenges for practitioners and service planners alike (Gray 1997);
◆ **new technology:** new technology is developing all the time. However,

such advances can lead to a high level of demand from specific populations (Gray 1997);

◆ **rising patient and professional expectations:** patient and professional expectations of health care are increasing. The new health-care 'consumers' expect more from services and are more prepared to invoke litigation and to take advantage of the educational opportunities afforded by new technologies, such as the Internet, in order to meet these expectations (Gray 1997).

These factors then represent some of the contexts which community-based practitioners must recognize if they are to be part of the attempt to drive health services away from the traditional and textbook approaches to decision making and towards finding the best available research evidence for decisions or treatment.

PROMOTING CLINICAL EFFECTIVENESS – DOING MORE GOOD THAN HARM

The term 'evidence-based health care' is often used to describe initiatives promoting clinical effectiveness. However, it also possesses a more specific sense, involving five key steps (Box 10.1).

Evidence-based health care (as expressed in these five broad steps) is simply about applying the best available research evidence to decision making. Such approaches to decision making are a means of improving the performance of all health professionals by making their practice more clinically effective and efficient. However, such approaches will fail if the three essential ingredients necessary for evidence-based health care are missing (Box 10.2).

The research evidence

Given that there are over two million articles published annually in over

---

Box 10.1 The five stages of an evidence-based approach to health care

◆ Identifying and refining a health care question/problem.

◆ Undertaking a comprehensive search of the relevant health care literature via electronic databases and hand-searching of references.

◆ Critically appraising each of the identified studies for quality and relevance.

◆ Interpreting the results of the data synthesis and making decisions about health care interventions.

◆ Evaluating performance.

Box 10.2 The essential ingredients for evidence-based health care

◆ High-quality, valid research evidence
◆ Making the research evidence available (dissemination)
◆ Acting on the evidence (implementation)

---

20 000 biomedical journals (Mulrow 1995), it is hardly surprising that health-care professionals find it increasingly difficult to keep abreast of all the available research relevant to their area of practice. The picture is complicated further when one considers the multiple types of study design which count as sources of research evidence. Not all designs are created equal, however, and the reader needs to be sure of the validity and appropriateness of the 'evidence' in relation to the health care questions being asked.

Randomized controlled trials

When assessing clinical effectiveness some designs are more valid than others because they are less prone to bias. Randomized controlled trials (RCTs), when done well, are the least susceptible to bias. Randomization of patients to treatments at the start of the trial will produce groups of patients who are identical in terms of factors such as disease severity and prognosis. If the treatment groups were unequally matched for prognosis and/or disease severity then the effect of the therapy could be exaggerated, cancelled or even counteracted (Sackett et al 1997).

Systematic reviews

Systematic reviews of research results provide the most reliable information on effectiveness (Chalmers & Altman 1995). They differ from more traditional literature reviews by the rigorous and systematic methods used to identify, quality appraise and include or exclude primary research results from the review. They are rigorous pieces of research in themselves which adhere to a strict methodological process.

> *A systematic review is the process of systematically locating, appraising and synthesizing research evidence from scientific studies in order to obtain a reliable overview.* (NHS Centre for Reviews and Dissemination 1996a)

Systematic reviews also pull together unmanageable amounts of research (NHS Centre for Reviews and Dissemination 1996a) which is an advantage for practitioners. A systematic review can be a review of studies which use similar designs, such as RCTs, or a review of studies using different research designs. The systematic review process involves several stages (Box 10.3).

Box 10.3 The systematic review process

◆ Identifying review questions
◆ Background research and problem specification
◆ Writing a review protocol
◆ Literature searching and study retrieval
◆ Assessing the relevance and validity of the studies
◆ Extracting data from primary studies
◆ Combining/summarizing the evidence
◆ Writing review report

(NHS Centre for Reviews and Dissemination 1996a)

For more detailed information regarding the process involved in undertaking a systematic review see the further reading suggestions at the end of this chapter.

Systematic reviews, like other research designs, vary in their quality and usefulness. A variety of checklists have been devised to assess the methodological quality of systematic reviews. An example of such a checklist is that used by the NHS Centre for Reviews and Dissemination (NHS CRD). At the NHS CRD, identified systematic reviews are appraised for quality before they are included on a Database of (good-quality) Abstracts of Reviews of Effectiveness (DARE) (see Boxes 10.6 and 10.7). For systematic reviews to be included on this database they have to meet four out of seven quality criteria.

◆ **Does the review have a clear question?** Ideally, a good review will have a well-defined question with clear objectives that include the following three components: target population; health-care intervention; outcomes of interest.
◆ **Does the review have a comprehensive search strategy?** A review must demonstrate that substantial effort to search for all relevant literature has been made. This will include details of sources searched (by electronic as well as traditional, hand-search means) and the key words used in those searches.
◆ **Does the review have any inclusion/exclusion criteria?** If inclusion/exclusion criteria are reported, are they appropriate? A good-quality review will have well-explained inclusion and exclusion criteria and these criteria will have been applied by more than one reviewer.
◆ **Has the validity of the studies been assessed?** A good-quality review is one where the validity of individual studies is assessed systematically, preferably by two reviewers.

◆ **Is sufficient detail of individual studies presented?** Details of individual studies are adequately presented in tables. Details may include:
   Study design
   Sample size in each study group
   Patient characteristics
   Interventions
   Settings
   Outcome measure
   Follow-up
   Drop-out rate
   Efficacious results
   Side-effects.
◆ **Is enough information given in the review to judge whether the author's summary and conclusion are appropriate?** (Song 1996)
◆ **How have the results been combined?** (either qualitatively or quantitatively) A good-quality review will·demonstrate appropriate combining or summaries of studies (Song 1996).

Other designs

Other study designs such as cohort studies, surveys and more qualitative research designs give valuable information and can be used in conjunction with RCTs to collect more qualitative information. This might include factors such as the impact of the intervention on subjects' families or carers, the experience of taking part in the study itself and the 'mapping' of contextual information relevant to the interpretation of the study's findings.

Dissemination

Effective dissemination is an essential prerequisite if action is to be based on research evidence. Dissemination ideally involves the targeted distribution of research information in appropriate formats to all relevant audiences. The current NHS R&D programme recognized early in its development that it is insufficient to simply fund research and not actively distribute the results and help ensure their adoption. This recognition led to the establishment of the Information Systems Strategy (ISS).

The information systems strategy

The ISS is about making research-based information available to health-care purchasers, providers, managers and policy makers. The ISS consists of:

◆ The National Research Register (NRR);
◆ The UK Cochrane Centre;
◆ The NHS Centre for Reviews and Dissemination (NHS CRD).

The National Research Register (formerly known as the Project Register System) is a register of ongoing research funded by the Department of Health and the NHS R&D programme. It also includes details of NHS-relevant, ongoing and future work funded by bodies such as the Medical Research Council. Box 10.4 explains how the reader can access information from the National Research Register.

The UK Cochrane Centre was established in 1992 as part of the ISS to facilitate and coordinate systematic up-to-date reviews of RCTs of the effects of health care (Mulrow & Oxman 1997). The UK Cochrane Centre is one of several international Cochrane Centres around the world coordinating the work of the Cochrane Collaboration. Nationally, it is a sibling centre to the NHS Centre for Reviews and Dissemination and the two collaborate closely in the production and dissemination of systematic reviews. The UK Cochrane Centre also manages the production of the Cochrane Library (Box 10.5).

The Cochrane Library is an excellent collection of high-quality review evidence on the effects of health care. Although currently stronger in some subjects than others, it is growing rapidly and can be a time-saving way of locating current effectiveness information. The Cochrane Library also contains details of how to undertake systematic reviews and information on the Cochrane Collaboration. Box 10.6 explains how the reader can access the Cochrane Library.

Box 10.4 The National Research Register (NRR)

◆ **How can the reader access information from the NRR?**
A public version of the NRR is available in all medical libraries.

◆ **Where can the reader learn more about it?**
The Research & Development Directorate, NHS Executive Headquarters, Quarry House, Quarry Hill, LEEDS LS2 7UE

Box 10.5 The Cochrane Library

The Cochrane Library is available on CD-ROM and contains four main databases:

◆ The Cochrane Database of Systematic Reviews (CDSR)
◆ The Database of Abstracts of Reviews of Effectiveness (DARE)
◆ The Cochrane Controlled Trials Register (CCTR)
◆ A methodology database

Box 10.6 Accessing the Cochrane Library

The Cochrane Database of Systematic Reviews (CDSR)
CDSR contains the full text of completed systematic reviews prepared by the Cochrane Collaboration as well as protocols for ongoing reviews.

The Database of Abstracts of Reviews of Effectiveness (DARE)
DARE contains critical assessments of good-quality systematic reviews. The systematic reviews abstracted for this database have been identified through the searching of international databases. Identified reviews are quality appraised for inclusion on the database by staff at the NHS CRD. The database also contains brief records of selected older reviews.

The Cochrane Controlled Trials Register (CCTR)
CCTR is a bibliography of controlled trials that have been identified by contributors to the Cochrane Collaboration.

How to access the Cochrane Library
The Cochrane Library is widely available in medical libraries. Personal copies can be purchased from Update Software Ltd, Summertown Pavilion Middle Way, Summertown, Oxford OX2 7LG, UK. Tel: +44 (0) 1865 513902. Fax: +44 (0) 1865 516918.
Web site: http://www.cochrane.co.uk
Email: info@update.co.uk

The NHS Centre for Reviews and Dissemination (NHS CRD) was established in 1994 and has three principal functions:

◆ carrying out and commissioning systematic reviews of the research literature on the effectiveness and cost-effectiveness of health-care interventions;
◆ maintaining the Database of Abstracts of Reviews of Effectiveness (DARE) and the NHS Economic Evaluation Database (Box 10.7);
◆ disseminating the results of good-quality reviews to the NHS and users of its services.

DARE contains abstracts of high-quality systematic review articles across the full range of health topics which have been identified and assessed by the review team at the NHS CRD. The systematic reviews abstracted for DARE are identified through searching international databases (MEDLINE, CINAHL and AMED). References and abstracts identified by a comprehensive search strategy are sifted by members of the CRD review team to identify published systematic reviews of effectiveness research. A second reviewer, blind to the results of the first, sifts references and abstracts again in the same way, thereby ensuring reliability in inclusion.

Identified reviews of effectiveness are then put through a second sifting

Box 10.7 The NHS Centre for Reviews and Dissemination Databases

How to access DARE

DARE can be accessed through:

◆ The Cochrane Library (see Box 10.6). This is available on CD-ROM and is updated quarterly.

◆ The WorldWide Web (and with Telnet enabled):http://www.york. ac.uk/inst/crd/info.htm. If prompted, the username and password are both: crduser.

◆ Telnet. Telnet to nhscrd.york.ac.uk: The username and password are both: crduser.

◆ Direct dial with a modem. Tel: +44 (0) 1904 431732. The username and password are both: crduser.

How to access NHS Economic Evaluation Database

The database may be accessed as for DARE. Both DARE and the NHS Economic Evaluation Databases can be accessed via the Information Service at CRD. This service is available to health-care professionals, commissioners, policy makers, providers and researchers when the enquirer has no other access to DARE or the NHS Economic Evaluation Database. Tel: +44 (0) 1904 433707. Fax: +44 (0) 1904 433661. Email: revdis@york.ac.uk.

process and examined for quality by two more reviewers. At this stage each reviewer, again blind to the other, applies a set of quality criteria to each of the identified reviews (as discussed on p. 201–202). Only those reviews that meet four or more of the six quality criteria are abstracted for DARE. Structured abstracts are written that allow an assessment of the strengths and weaknesses of the systematic review and include, where possible, clinical implications and a critical commentary.

The NHS Economic Evaluation Database contains abstracts of economic evaluations of health-care interventions. Evaluations such as cost-benefit analyses and cost-effectiveness analyses are identified from international databases and detailed structured abstracts written by health economists. The abstracts comment on the methodology, results and conclusions of the studies.

The NHS Economic Evaluation Database and DARE are available to the whole health-care community free of charge. For information about how to access these databases, see Box 10.7.

In addition to working with the electronic medium of the Internet, NHS CRD produces the dissemination products Effective Health Care Bulletins, Effectiveness Matters and CRD Reports.

Effective Health Care Bulletins are 8–12-page summaries of the results of a systematic review of the acceptability, clinical (and cost) effectiveness of particular health service interventions. The bulletins are aimed at health-care purchasers and providers and are written in language that can be understood by people without clinical training. They are normally based on the results of a systematic review undertaken or commissioned by NHS CRD. Details about Effective Health Care Bulletins can be obtained from the Publications Office at NHS CRD.

Effectiveness Matters are summaries of the best available research evidence in specific areas of effectiveness. This research evidence is based on systematic reviews or large-scale, high-quality RCTs which have been carried out by research teams outside the NHS CRD but which have important messages. Again, these are written in language easily understandable to people without clinical training. If anything, the style is even more accessible to members of the public than the Effective Health Care Bulletin. Contact the Publications Office, NHS CRD, University of York, York YO1 5DD (+44 (0) 1904 433648) for further details.

CRD Reports provide a full and detailed write-up of systematic reviews and other research undertaken or commissioned by NHS CRD. These can be obtained from the publications office above.

NURSING AND THE NHS RESEARCH AND DEVELOPMENT STRATEGY

In response to the NHS R&D programme a taskforce was established to consider the role, potential and future development of research in nursing, midwifery and health visiting (Department of Health 1993). The report of the taskforce represents a means of ensuring that research in these professions makes a full and integrated contribution to the pursuit of health gain. Recommendation 31 of the taskforce report states:

> We recommend that when the Review Commissioning Facility (NHS CRD) is established a nursing and midwifery dimension should be built into their programme and that they be commissioned to undertake and publish regular critical overviews of research in specific fields. (Department of Health 1993)

One of the ways in which this particular recommendation was taken forward was with the establishment of the Practice and Service Development Initiative (PSDI) within the NHS CRD.

The Practice and Service Development Initiative

The Practice and Service Development Initiative was established to identify and document existing practice and service developments within the nursing and therapy professions throughout the UK. From this examination the project identified the key health care professionals involved in these developments. A broad range of health care professionals were covered including therapists, nurses and midwives.

Practice and service development information gathered from health care professionals identified topic areas where practice and service development activity is most common. The research evidence behind those topic areas with a high level of development activity was ascertained and disseminated. Where there was no good-quality review information but substantive primary research in a topic area, the project informed the NHS CRD management team who in turn inform those with responsibility for commissioning systematic reviews. Where there was no (good-quality) primary research information in a topic area of high-level development activity, then again the NHS CRD management team informed the National R&D agenda of the need for more research in these areas.

WHAT CAN NURSES DO?

In order to implement evidence-based health care in the community, nurses are expected to identify the best available research evidence for specific health-care problems and apply that evidence in daily practice. Using the five basic steps outlined in Box 10.1 it is possible to see how nurses might utilize an evidence-based approach with the aid of a few examples.

An example – school nurses and teenage pregnancies

A school nurse may wish to find out about the latest research evidence on preventing teenage pregnancies because she has been wondering whether or not it would be useful to implement a school-based programme of education for teenagers on the subject of contraceptive use.

Step 1   Identify and refine the question

Q. Are school education programmes on the use of contraceptives effective?

A quick background search of the literature helps refine the question. For example, it helps the school nurse to decide whether to look solely at contraceptive use or whether to include prevention of teenage pregnancy and/or the treatment of unwanted pregnancy. The search also helps clarify the specific age range of the client group. So the refined question might look something like this.

Q. Are education programmes for 10–12-year-olds on the use of contraceptives effective in reducing rates of teenage pregnancy?

Step 2   The search

Once the question is clear a search of electronic databases is undertaken. For this, the nurse needs access to library facilities and the skills to design a comprehensive search strategy. If the nurse does not possess these skills then the local librarian should be able to assist. Example search strategies are available from NHS CRD (NHS Centre for Reviews and Dissemination 1996a).

Step 3   Critical appraisal and data synthesis

Once all studies on the topic have been identified and selected for inclusion, the school nurse critically appraises each of the studies for quality. She then abstracts the data from each of the included studies, synthesizes and analyses them. Organizations such as NHS CRD and the Cochrane Collaboration can give valuable insight into the processes involved.

Step 4   Implementation

Before any research findings can be applied to practice, one needs to interpret the results and assess whether or not the findings can be generalized and applied to the school nurse's particular environment. Specific environments pose specific challenges. For example, the nurse working with young people with special educational needs may find that applying the findings of a review of the research evidence focusing on a general population of 10–18-year-olds is inappropriate.

Step 5   Evaluation

If the results of the research are applied then they will also need to be evaluated. The nurse might wish to contact her local clinical audit group and develop a series of audit protocols in conjunction with other colleagues such as local general practitioners or teachers.

Practicalities

The above example of an evidence-based approach is something of a 'purist's' approach and may prove impractical. For example, practitioners may lack one or more of the prerequisite skills, resources or knowledge to successfully apply it 'wholesale'. This does not mean, however, that the basic techniques are irrelevant and cannot be adopted in more applied ways. Community nurses (and other professionals) involved in health care, health education and promotion rarely have the time, resources or skills to search and critically appraise all relevant research in an effort to identify the best evidence to inform their practice (Droogan & Song 1996). An alternative approach is to have steps 2 and 3 undertaken by people who have the appropriate skills. The Information Systems Strategy, mentioned earlier, provides health-care providers, commissioners, managers and policy makers with information resources based on steps 2 and 3.

The resources listed in Boxes 10.6 and 10.7 provide nurses with good-quality systematically reviewed information, as do Effective Health Care Bulletins and Effectiveness Matters. These tangible outputs from the ISS (Box 10.8) are available to all health-care professionals and alleviate the need for health-care professionals to be experts in areas such as search strategy development, data analysis, critical appraisal and clinical practice. They leave health-care professionals free to concentrate on getting the best available research evidence into clinical practice. It is worth highlighting how these 'evidence-based shortcuts' might work in practice.

Example One   Using an Effective Health Care Bulletin to impact on service delivery

Using the previous example of the school nurse and the question: 'Are education programmes for 10–12-year-olds on the use of contraceptives effective in reducing rates of teenage pregnancy?', the Effective Health Care Bulletin on Teenage Pregnancy (NHS Centre for Reviews and Dissemination 1997) could save the school nurse a great deal of time. This particular bulletin summarizes the research evidence in the area of preventing and reducing the adverse

---

Box 10.8 Access to other evidence-based health-care information

Evidence-based nursing
The Evidence-Based Nursing Journal is published jointly by the BMJ Publishing Group and the RCN Publishing Company. This journal identifies and summarizes primary research and review articles that are of a high quality. Each article is followed by a brief, expert commentary on the context of each article.

For more information contact: Subscriptions Department, RCN Publishing Company, Glynteg House, Station Terrace, Cardiff CF5 4XG, UK. Tel: +44 (0) 1222 576208. Fax: +44 (0) 1222 553411.

Bandolier
This is an eight-sided monthly issue distributed free of charge within the NHS. It contains short articles which summarize and discuss important evidence, explanations of statistical procedures and other issues relating to evidence-based health care. It is produced by Anglia and Oxford Regional Health Authority. For more information contact: Dr R A Moore, Dr H McQuay, Dr J A Muir Gray, Bandolier Editorial Office, c/o Pain Relief Unit, The Churchill, Oxford OX3 7LJ.

effects of unintended teenage pregnancies. The bulletin states as one of its key findings that:

> *School-based sex education can be effective in reducing teenage pregnancy, especially when linked to access to contraceptive services. The most reliable evidence shows that it does not increase sexual activity or pregnancy rates.* (NHS Centre for Reviews and Dissemination 1997)

By using this Effective Health Care Bulletin, the nurse has found the answer to her question without having to commit herself to time-consuming research identification, retrieval and appraisal. Moreover, she can be confident about the quality of the evidence and the messages she is applying.

Example Two   Effectiveness Matters

This example shows how a different dissemination product, Effectiveness Matters (EM), might influence evidence-based health care for older clients of the community practitioner. The October 1996 issue of EM – Influenza Vaccination and Older People – was a critical summary of the research evidence in this area and stated that:

> *Annual influenza vaccination of all older people (over 65 years) is a cost-effective way of reducing influenza-related deaths in illness.* (NHS Centre for Reviews and Dissemination 1996b)

Current health-care policy on this issue recommends that only 'at-risk' patients (patients with angina or chronic respiratory problems) over the age of 65 years should be vaccinated. Yet the research evidence shows that:

> *Influenza vaccination is a cost-effective way of reducing morbidity and saving lives in people over 65 ...* (NHS Centre for Reviews and Dissemination 1996b)

Vaccination of all older people, rather than those in high-risk groups, offers greater potential to reduce admissions to hospital for influenza-related illnesses such as respiratory problems and pneumonia.

Clearly the community nurse in receipt of this information is in a position to influence other members of the primary health-care team and to steer the development of multidisciplinary strategies to implement these findings locally.

DOES NURSING HAVE ANY RESEARCH EVIDENCE?

A common misconception is that nursing does not have good-quality evaluative research in the form of systematic reviews and RCTs to draw on. This is often based on the premise that nursing itself cannot be subjected to such rigorous research designs. This is not the case. Droogan & Cullum (1998) set out to identify systematic reviews relevant to nursing, the aim being to:

◆ identify systematic reviews of effectiveness in areas of nursing practice;
◆ describe the identified systematic reviews in terms of the aspects of nursing covered and the quality of the reviews;
◆ make the most recent systematic reviews of effectiveness in nursing accessible by including them in DARE.

A combination of MEDLINE searching (1987–1994), hand-searching of nursing journals from inception to 1994 and informal contact with nurse researchers in the UK and abroad identified 81 papers for further scrutiny. On examination, 36 of the 81 papers were reviews which addressed questions of effectiveness. These were quality appraised using NHS early CRD quality criteria, namely:

◆ Does the review have a well-defined question?
◆ Does the review demonstrate a comprehensive search strategy?
◆ Is data synthesis appropriate?

Of the 36 reviews extracted, 53% (19) of them met all three quality criteria and were subsequently included on DARE (Droogan & Cullum 1998). The identified reviews were in key clinical areas for community nurses, including palliative care, patient education and leg ulcer management.

In an earlier work Cullum (1997) investigated the extent of RCTs which were of direct relevance to nursing. This was undertaken as part of the development of a nursing contribution to the Cochrane Collaboration. Through searching MEDLINE (1966–1994) and the hand-searching of 11 nursing research journals (from inception to 1994) more than 500 RCTs were identified, a process which is continuing. Once again these studies were in key nursing topic areas (Box 10.9).

Both of these pieces of work negate the oft-quoted complaint that there

---

Box 10.9 Examples of nursing topic areas with RCT evidence to support interventions

Patient education	Midwifery or neonatal care
Nurse education	Cardiac rehabilitation
Postoperative care	Anxiety prevention or reduction
Pain	Preoperative care
Paediatric nursing	Health promotion
	(Cullum 1997)

are no RCTs and systematic reviews relevant to nursing. Moreover, they also show that rigorous research designs have been and can be applied to nursing research on effectiveness. However, there are still many areas of nursing where more rigorous primary research is required, including the arena of community practice. Community nurses have a professional obligation to base practice on the best available research evidence but more than this, they also should strive to contribute to the primary research knowledge base. They can do this by publishing and disseminating their evaluations of evidence-based practice but also by playing an active part in local and national primary research projects.

CONCLUSION

Health care is a multiprofessional and multidisciplinary collaborative project and community nurses need to play a full and active role in the primary-care team if they wish to deliver practice which is both clinically effective and efficient. However, this role and the evaluation which accompanies it need to be based on something a little more substantive than tradition or 'gut feelings' about nursing practice. The shift to evidence-based practice offers nurses the chance to base their work in the team on something which is 'transparent' to other professionals, colleagues and service users alike.

An evidence-based approach to health care has three key stages:

◆ creating the research evidence;
◆ making the research evidence available;
◆ acting on the evidence.

The importance of these is evident throughout this chapter. Knowing where to access the research evidence is very important because there is such a huge volume of information available to health-care professionals, albeit of varying types and quality. As Sheldon & Melville (1996) point out, when health-care professionals are keen to:

> ... reflect on their practice and try to increase the clinical effectiveness of the services they provide, they are faced with the question of where to get the information from.

As a key part of these reflections, systematic reviews of research evidence and RCT evidence itself provide the most reliable sources of information on effectiveness. The identification and dissemination of good-quality evidence is made much easier through the work of the Cochrane Collaboration and the NHS Centre for Reviews and Dissemination. Practitioners now have access to reliable and, perhaps equally importantly, 'trustworthy' evidence.

The single most important theme of this chapter has been the demystification of evidence-based health care for the community nurse. If it helps point this key member of the primary health team in the direction of research evidence to inform their practice, then it will have served its purpose. If evidence-based health care is to permeate down to the level of community nurses then nurse educators, textbooks and continuing education programmes must introduce the key elements of the approach. These include: the systematic review and RCT as a research design; critical appraisal skills; seeking and using sources of high-quality research evidence. Just as important, however, is the 'building in' of the evidence-based message to all levels of evaluation in services:

◆ the individual practitioner: perhaps through an evidence-based component in reflections on practice and/or clinical supervision;
◆ the service: through strategic commissioning of local clinical audits;
◆ the organization: through the implementation and adaptation of guidelines and protocols and appropriate involvement with the work of the Department of Health and the Royal Colleges.

Nursing is in a better position now than it has ever been to take up the challenge of building and shaping evidence-based cultures at all levels of the NHS machine.

QUESTIONS FOR DISCUSSION

◆ Think of a clinical question or problem that you may have at present and discuss how you might go about finding an evidence-based answer to the question/problem.

◆ Discuss what changes to practice you might make and the problems you might encounter in implementation and evaluation of any likely changes.

ANNOTATED BIBLIOGRAPHY

NHS Centre for Reviews and Dissemination 1996 Undertaking systematic reviews of research on effectiveness. CRD guidelines for those carrying out or commissioning reviews. NHS Centre for Reviews and Dissemination, York

A well-written, readable, concise yet relatively comprehensive text on how to undertake a systematic review.

Droogan J, Song F 1996 The process and importance of systematic reviews. Nurse Researcher 4 (1)

A more nurse-specific, brief overview of the systematic review process.

Sackett D L, Richardson W S, Rosenberg W, Haynes R B 1997 Evidence-based medicine. How to practice and teach EBM. Churchill Livingstone, London

An excellent book on how to teach evidence-based medicine.

Entwistle V, Watt I S, Herring J E 1996 Information about health-care effectiveness. King's Fund Publishing, London

An introduction to the theory and practice surrounding the evidence-based approach to health care.

Acknowledgements

Professor Ian Watt, Dr Vikki Entwistle and Julie Glanville provided helpful suggestions and comments.

REFERENCES

Chalmers I, Altman D G (eds) 1995 Systematic reviews. BMJ Publishing, London

Cullum N 1997 The identification and analysis of randomised controlled trials in nursing: a preliminary study. Quality In Health Care 6: 1–5

Department of Health 1993 Report of the taskforce on the strategy for research in nursing, midwifery and health visiting. Department of Health, London

Droogan J, Cullum N 1998 Systematic reviews. International Journal of Nursing Studies 35 (1): 13–22

Droogan J, Song F 1996 The process and importance of systematic reviews. Nurse Researcher 4 (1): 15–26

Entwistle V, Watt I S, Herring J E 1996 Information about health-care effectiveness. King's Fund Publishing, London

Gray J A M 1997 Evidence-based healthcare. How to make health policy and management decisions. Churchill Livingstone, London

Mulrow C D 1995 Rationale for systematic reviews. In: Chalmers I, Altman D G (eds) Systematic reviews. BMJ Publishing, London

Mulrow C D, Oxman A D (eds) Cochrane Collaboration Handbook (updated 1 March 1997). In: The Cochrane Library [Database on disk and CD-ROM]. The Cochrane Collaboration, Oxford

NHS Centre for Reviews and Dissemination 1996a Undertaking systematic reviews of research on effectiveness: CRD guidelines for those carrying out or commissioning reviews. NHS Centre for Reviews and Dissemination, York

NHS Centre for Reviews and Dissemination 1996b Influenza vaccination and older people. Effectiveness Matters 2 (1): 1–4

NHS Centre for Reviews and Dissemination 1997 Preventing and reducing the adverse effects of unintended teenage pregnancies. Effective Health-Care Bulletin 3 (1): 1–12

Sackett D L, Richardson W S, Rosenberg W A, Haynes R B 1997 Evidence-based medicine. How to practice and teach EBM. Churchill Livingstone, London

Sheldon T, Melville A 1996 Providing intelligence for rational decision-making in the NHS: The NHS Centre for Reviews and Dissemination. Journal of clinical effectiveness 1 (2): 51–54

Song F 1996 Checklist for quality assessment of published reviews. NHS Centre for Reviews and Dissemination, York (unpublished)

Index

Location references in bold indicate figures and tables

A

Accident and Emergency departments, nursing developments, 185
Advocacy
  disabled people, 165
  minority groups, 32
Arenas, defining, 9, 10
Asians *see* South Asians
Assessing needs, school nursing, 84–86, 88–89, 92–93, 98
Audit commission, 6
Audit Commission report, *Making a Reality of Community Care*, 159

B

Bandolier, 209
Bradford University School of Health Studies, recruitment practice evaluation, 24, 37–38
British Medical Association, definitions of skill mix, 49

C

Career, practice nursing as, 139, 140, 147–148
Caring for People, White Paper, 1989, 159–160
Caseloads
  see also Workload
  CPNs, 114, 116, 123, 125
  school nurses, 83
Chief nursing officer (CNO), 156
Child health surveillance, 84, 88–89
  evaluating, 100–101
Children
  health needs, 85
    assessing, 84–86, 88–89, 92–93, 98
  as service users, 86–87, 89–90, 101, 103
The Children Act, 1989, 86
Choice and Opportunity, White Paper, 1996, 61–62
Clinical effectiveness, promoting, 199–206
  research evidence, 199–202
    dissemination, 202–206
Cochrane Library, 203
  accessing, 204
Code of Professional Conduct, UKCC 1992, 27, 154
Communication and language barriers, 31–33
Community care
  definitions and concept, 158–159
  impact of increased, 184
  mentally ill, move towards, 111
  multidisciplinary working, 190
  principal elements, 157
  provision of services, 160–161

Community mental health team (CMHT), 111
  see also Community psychiatric nursing
  authority and responsibility, 125
  discord within, 118–119, 125–126
Community nurses
  competence, identification and examination, 174–175
  and evidence-based practice, 212
Community nursing
  environmental factors, care delivery, 174
  isolated nature of, 184
  provision, 4–7
  roles, changing, 5
    enhanced *see* Role extension and enhancement
Community psychiatric nursing, 107–126
  background history, 108
  and chronic mental illness, 121–122
  clients
    accepting, 114–116, 123, 125
    discharging, 117–118, 123, 124, 125
    referrals, 112, 113–114, 116, 119
  clinical autonomy, 107–108, 112, 122
    managerial negligence, 123
  discussions with colleagues, 116–117
  expectations of referrer, 113–114
  psychiatrists, resisting dominance of, 119–120, 125–126
  questions for discussion, 126
  rigour in practice, need for, 123–125
  role of CPNs, 121–122, 125
  role, performance and status study
    aims, 108–109
    context of study, 109–111
    discussion, 122–125
    findings, 112–122
    methods, 111–112
  supervision, 120–121, 124–125, 125
Community service provision, learning disabilities
  evaluation, 164–165, 166–167
  residential systems, 166
Competences
  best settings in which to observe specific, 178, **181–182**
  groups observed, 178–179, **180**
  in institutional and community settings, 190–191
  moving from institutional care into home care, 183–184
  specific nursing skills, 185–188
Competences, mapping changing, 171–196
  care settings, skills and competences, 178–190
  competence and evaluation, conceptual link, 171–172
  competence identification and examination methodology, community nurses, 174–175
  questions for discussion, 191

Competences, mapping changing (*contd*)
  study
    aims, 172
    competence groups, constituents,
      192–196
    findings, 177–178
    methods used, 176–177
Context of care, 174, 183–184
Continuity of care, community nurses,
    187–188
Cost
  consciousness, learning disabilities services,
    161
  effectiveness, nurse prescribing, 68–69
Court Report, DHSS 1976, 83
CRD Reports, 206
Crown Report, DoH 1989a, 66–67, 68, 70, 71
Cultural diversities in health care, 23–40
  see also Ethnic minorities
  community nursing in multiracial Britain,
    24–37
  equal opportunities and nurse recruitment,
    37–38
  questions for discussion, 39–40
Culturally diverse
  populations, community nurses working
    within, 27
  workforce, need for, 24
Culture
  and behaviour patterns, overemphasis, 28
  interpreting differences as deviance, 29–30
  role in health care, 27–29
Culyer Report, 7
Cumberlege Report, DHSS 1986, 65–66
Cybersociety, 109

D

Database of Abstracts of Reviews of
    Effectiveness (DARE), 201–202, 204–205
Delegation
  GPs to practice nurses, 137–138
  skill mix in PCHTs, 50–53, 60–61
  study, 56–57, 57–59
Delivering the Future, DoH 1996a, 61–62, 72
*Developing the Role of the District Nurse in the
    Administration of Intravenous Therapy in
    the Home*, ENB 1994, 188
Diagnosing, nurse prescribing, 70
Disabled people
  see also Learning disability
  care, historical dimension, 155–156
  empowerment, 154
Disadvantaged groups and service provision,
    26–27
Dissemination, research evidence, 202–206
District nurses
  technical nature of care, 187–188
  workload, 55, 59–60
Drop-in sessions, school nurses, 90, 91

E

Education Acts, 81–82
Education and preparation
  see also Competences, mapping changing
  community mental health staff, 110
  for multiethnic clientele, 38–39
  practice nursing, 133–134, 142–143
  prescribing, 67–68, 71–73
  school nursing, 97–99
Effective Health-care Bulletins, 206
  example of use, 209–210
Effectiveness Matters, 206
  example of use, 210
English National Board (ENB), district nurses,
    developing role, 188
Enhanced roles, 58, 185–188
  and boundary definitions, 46–47
Equal opportunities and nurse recruitment, 37–38
Ethnic minorities, 7, 24–25
  assumptions based on sterotypes, 28
  communication and language barriers, 31–33
  disadvantaged groups and community care
    services, 26–27
  identifying health needs, 25–27
  insensitive and inappropriate care, 30–31
  interpreting differences as deviance, 29–30
  and nurse recruitment, 24, 37–38
  nurse tutors, underepresentation, 38–39
  and nursing, 33, 35–36
  resident population by ethnic group, **25**
*Ethnic Minority Staff in the NHS: A Programme
    of Action*, DoH 1993, 33, 34
Evaluation
  and community nursing, 8–17
    policy and practice, 9–12
  different aspects, example, 11
  and evidence-based practice, 7
  models available, 12, 13
  reasons for in nursing, 12–14
Evidence-based approach, 7
  see also Research evidence
  and the community practitioner, 197–213
    NHS research and development strategy,
      206–207
    promoting clinical effectiveness, 199–206
  questions for discussion, 213
  essential ingredients, 200
  five stages, 199
  information, access to, 204, 205, 209
  key stages, 212
  school nursing, 99–100
  shift towards, factors influencing, 198–199
  use by nurses, 207–210
Evidence-Based Nursing Journal, 209

F

FHSA
  nurse advisors supporting nurses, 142–143

FHSA (*contd*)
  reimbursement of practice staff costs,
    131–132
Five stages of evidence-based approach, 199
Focus group, 176
Focus group discussions, delegation, 57–58
Fragmentation of care, 50, 52
Fulcher, model of policy levels and arenas, 9,
  10
Functional autonomy, Allport, 164
Funding for training, prescribing, 73

G

General practice
  fundholding, 46
  as organisational base of primary care, 4–5
  recruitment and retention crisis, 45, 46
General practitioners
  contracts, 12, 52, 71
    and growth of practice nursing, 131
  employment and management of practice
    nurses, 148
    tasks expected to undertake, **52**
Georgian Society pilot study, 51
Greenhalgh Report, 1994, 185–186

H

Health commissioners, 6–7
  and practice nursing, 143–144
  school nursing, 85
Health education, school nursing, 87
  sex education, 94
Health of the Nation, DoH 1992, 7, 26, 87, 93
Health needs
  children, 84–86, 88–89, 92–93, 98
  ethnic minorities, 25–27
Health patterns, ethnic minorities, 25
  targeting screening programmes, 29
Health promotion
  move towards, 7
  school nursing, 87, 93–95, 98
    mental health, 94
Health surveillance, school nursing, 84, 88–89
  evaluation, 100–101
Health visitors
  prescribing, 69
  workload, 59–60
    skill mix study, 55–56
Health of the Young Nation, DoH 1995, 87
Health care
  interviews, school nurses, 89, 89–90
  rising expectations of, 199
Homicide, schizophrenic perpetrators, 123,
  124
Hospital setting, multidisciplinary working,
  188–190

I

Immunization programmes, school nursing, 84
Information, ethnic minorities, access to, 32
Information systems strategy, 202–206,
  208–209
Institutional discrimination, 29
The Interface between the Doctor and Other
  Members of the Primary Health–Care
  Team, DOH study, 49, 53–59
Internal market, 6, 46
Internet addiction, 109
Interpreters, 32
Interprofessional working *see* Multidisciplinary
  working
Interview approach, qualitative methodology,
  137
  semistructured interview, 176

J

Jay Committee, 159
Junior hosiptal doctors, working hours
  reduction, 185, 186

L

Language barriers, communication, 31–33
Learning disability, 153–167
  challenges relating to health, 163
  contemporary service development,
    156–157
  general holistic needs of people with, 163
  historical dimension, 155–156
  nursing practice, contemporary statements
    relating to, 161–163
  policy development, 158–161
  prevelance of severe, 157
  professional reaction to change, 163–167
  questions for discussion, 167
  service provision changes, resistance,
    165–166
  specialist nurses, 162–163
Link workers, 32
Locus of responsibility, community-based
  residential systems, 166

M

Making a Reality of Community Care, Audit
  Commission report, 159
Managerialism, 6–7, 9
  in primary care, 146
  supervision, practice nursing, 141
Medical responsibility and CPNS, 119, 120
Medicinal Products Prescription by Nurses Act
  1992, 67
Medicine and nursing, redefinition of
  boundaries, 185

Mental health
 cultural context, 30
 young people, *94*
Mental Health Act 1959, 158
Mental health industry, 109–110
 nursing, role and direction, 110–111
Mental Health (Patients in the Community)
  Act, 1995, 124
Mental illness, CPNs and chronic, 121–122
Minority ethnic groups *see* Ethnic minorities
Models
 of competence, 171–172, **173**
 of evaluation, 12, 13
Multidisciplinary working, 188–190
 see also Community mental health team
  (CMHT)
Multiethnic workforce, need for, 24, 33

N

National Research Register, 203
Needs and priorities, 5–7
Needs-led service, school nursing, 84–87,
  88–93
 needs assessment, 84–86, 92–93, 98–99
A New Deal, DoH 1991, 185, 186
NHS Act 1977, medical and dental inspections,
  82
NHS Centre for Reviews and Dissemination
  (NHS CRD), 201, 204, 205
 reports, 206
NHS and Community Care Act 1990, 26, 88,
  156–157, 159, 160
NHS Economic Evaluation Database, 205
NHS, internal market, 6
NHS research and development strategy,
  206–207
NHS trusts and practice nursing, 143–144
Night practitioner's role, 186
Nurse practitioner, 47, 66
 see also Prescribing
 competences and extended roles, 186–187
 GP's views of role, 145
 prescribing, 58–59
Nurse Prescribers' Formulary (NPF), 68
Nurse prescribing *see* Prescribing
Nurse recruitment
 equal opportunities and development project,
  37–38
 from ethnic minorities, 33, 35–38
Nurse training *see* Education and preparation
Nurse tutors, underrepresentation of ethnic
  minorities, 38–39
Nurses in hospital-based multidisciplinary
  teams, 190
Nursing
 and ethnic minority groups, 33, 35–36,
  38–39
 new professional groups within, 46–47
 research evidence relevant to, 210–212

role, extension and enhancement, 46–47, 58,
  185–188
Nursing, midwifery and health visiting staff by
  age and ethnic group, **35**

O

*Opportunities for Change: A New Direction
 for Nursing for People with Learning
 Disabilities*, 1993 conference, 161–162

P

Parental control of children's health, 90
Patient's Charter, 26
 Services for Children and Young People,
  86–87, 101
Pluralist approach, evaluation, 136
Policy
 context of school nursing, 84–88
 goals, school nurses working within, 102
 levels and arenas in NHS, 9, **10**
 and practice
  contested domains, 10–12
  evaluating, 9–12
 in welfare provision, 6–7
Population ageing, 198
Post registration education and practice (PREP),
  73
Post registration level training, school nurses,
  97–98
Practice nurse
 cost-effectiveness, 133
 education and preparation, 72, 133–134,
  142–143
 enhanced roles, 46–47, 71
 organisation of work, 141–142
 reasons for becoming, 138–140
 variations in roles, 132–133
 workforce growth, 46
 workload, 59
  skill mix study, 55
  tasks expected to undertake, **52**
Practice nursing, emergence and development,
  129–149
 evaluating, 131
 policy context, 131–134
 questions for discussion, 148–149
 role in primary care, study, 134–147
  qualitative evaluation, 135–137
  research findings, 137–147
 stakeholders in, 134
Practice and Service Development Initiative,
  206–207
Practice, variations in, 197–198
Preparation and education *see* Education and
  preparation
Preregistration training, school nurses, 97
Prescribing
 by nurse practitioners, 58–59

Prescribing (*contd*)
  and community nursing, 65–74
  evaluation
    feasibility study, 67–68
    implications for practice and management, 73–74
    preparation, 71–73
    professional roles, 70–71
    service delivery, 68–69
  forms of, 66
  funding for training, 73
  GP's views, 58–59, 144–145
  Nurse Prescribers' Formulary (MPF), 68
  organizational changes, 67–68
  qualifications and eligibility, 71–73
  questions for discussion, 74
Primary care
  changes, 46–47
  development, 148
  shift from secondary care, 4–5, 88, 132
  skill mix in *see* Skill mix in primary care
Primary care-led NHS and school health, 88, 95–96
Primary health-care team
  defining, 49–**50**
  school nursing, potential for integrating, 96
Priorities and needs, 5–7
Professional
  accountability, 187
  power, 174
  roles, nurse prescribing, 70–71
  status, school nursing, 80
Profiling, school health, 89, 94, 103
Project 2000 registered nurse (child branch) diploma, 97
Project Register System *see* National Research Register
Psychiatrists and CPNs, 119–120, 125–126
  and CPNs role, 122
  discharge, 118
  referral system, 114
    and medical responsibility, 119–120

Q

Qualitative
  approaches, value of, 15–16
  techniques, 136–137
Qualitative and quantitative methodologies, 14–17, 175, 202
Quantitative approaches, value of, 16–17

R

Racism in nursing, 36
Randomised controlled trials, 200
  relevant to nursing, 211–212
Recruitment
  and ethnic minorities, 24, 33, 35–38
  and retention crisis, general practice, 45, 46

Research evidence
  dissemination, 202–206
  relevant to nursing, 210–212
  systematic reviews, 200–202
Research methodology
  focus group, 176
  qualitative approach, 15–16, 136–137, 175
  qualitative/quantitative approach, 14–17, 175, 202
  quantitative approach, 16–17
  randomised controlled trials, 200
  semistructured interviews, 137, 176
  triangulation, 175
Residential systems, community based, 166
Ritchie Report, 1994, 123
Role extension and enhancement, 58, 71, 185–188
  and boundary definitions, 46–47

S

Schizophrenic homicide rates, 124
School health profiling, 89, 94, 103
School health service, 81–83
  DoH objectives, 82
  functions, 83
  negotiating service level agreements, 91, 92
  in primary care-led NHS, 88, 95–96
  school nursing as part of, 79–80
  statutory requirements, 81–82
School nursing, 79–103
  access to pupils, 90–91
  caseloads, 83
  developing role, 98–99
  education and preparation for, 97–99
  evaluating services, 99–102
  health promotion, 87, 93–95, 98
  integration into PCHTs, 96
  involving service users, 86–87, 89–92, 103
    in evaluation, 101
  low profile and disinvestment, 79–80, 85
  policy
    context, 84–88
    developments and role of, 88–96
    goals, working within, 102
  potential, 92–93
  questions for discussion, 103
  role of, study, 80–81, 84, 93–95
  school as setting for nursing work, 95–96
  and teenage pregnancies, example of evidence-based practice, 207–208
  variations in practice, 85–86, 92
Scope of Professional Practice, UKCC 1992, 99, 185
Screening programmes, targeting ethnic minority groups, 29–30
Semistructured interviews, 137, 176
Service
  delivery, nurse prescribing, impact, 68–69

Service (*contd*)
  provision, organisation around white norms,
    29–30
Sex education, school nurse as teacher, 94
Skill mix, 5
  defining, 49
  school nursing teams, 93
Skill mix in primary care, 45–62
  agenda for scrutiny, 59–61
  questions for discussion, 62
  study, 49, 53–59
  understanding, 48–53
South Asians
  kinship relationships and networks, 29
  midwives stereotypical understanding of, 28
  recruitment and retention in health-care,
    research and development project,
    37–38
  underrepresentation in NHS, 24, 36–37
Stakeholders, evaluation of services, 10, 11, 12,
    131, 134
Stereotypes, assumptions based on, 28, 29
Systematic reviews
  relevant to nursing, 211
  of research results, 200–202

T

Technology, 198–199
  cybersociety, 109
  technical nature, care in the community,
    187–188
Touche Ross study, DoH 1991, 67, 68, 70
Training *see* Education and preparation
Triage
  nurses undertaking, 185
  in primary care, 47, 61
Triangulation, 175

U

UK Cochrane Centre, 203
UKCC
  Code of Professional Conduct, 154
    working in multicultural settings, 27
  postregistration education and practice,
    97–98
  practice nurse training, 72
  Scope of Professional Practice, 1992, 99, 185
United Nations Convention on the Rights of
    the Child, 86
University of York, enquiry into general
    practice recruitment and retention, 45
Uptake of services, ethnic minorities, 30–31

V

Value for Money report, 51
Variations in practice
  district and practice nurses, 197–198
  school nurses, 85–86, 92
Voluntary sector organisations
  care in the community, 184
  ethnic minorities, services for, 31

W

Workforce
  changes, NHS, 46
  culturally diverse, need for, 24, 33
  recruitment, 33, 35–38
    and retention crisis, 45, 46
Workload
  assessment, skill mix, 59–60
  changes in, 47
  management, skill mix in PCHTs, 48–49
  school nurses, 83
  skill mix study, 55–56